The
GLP-1
SOLUTION

175+ Strategies, Tips, and Tools to
Maximize Your Weight Loss and Feel Your
Best on Semaglutide, Tirzepatide, and More

GIANNA BEASLEY, RD

ADAMS MEDIA

New York   Amsterdam/Antwerp   London   Toronto   Sydney/Melbourne   New Delhi

Aadamsmedia
Adams Media
An Imprint of Simon & Schuster, LLC
100 Technology Center Drive
Stoughton, MA 02072

For more than 100 years, Simon & Schuster has championed authors and the stories they create. By respecting the copyright of an author's intellectual property, you enable Simon & Schuster and the author to continue publishing exceptional books for years to come. We thank you for supporting the author's copyright by purchasing an authorized edition of this book.

No amount of this book may be reproduced or stored in any format, nor may it be uploaded to any website, database, language-learning model, or other repository, retrieval, or artificial intelligence system without express permission. All rights reserved. Inquiries may be directed to Simon & Schuster, 1230 Avenue of the Americas, New York, NY 10020 or permissions@simonandschuster.com.

Copyright © 2025 by Simon & Schuster, LLC.

All rights reserved, including the right to reproduce this book or portions thereof in any form whatsoever. For information, address Adams Media Subsidiary Rights Department, 1230 Avenue of the Americas, New York, NY 10020.

First Adams Media trade paperback edition
September 2025

ADAMS MEDIA and colophon are registered trademarks of Simon & Schuster, LLC.

Simon & Schuster strongly believes in freedom of expression and stands against censorship in all its forms. For more information, visit BooksBelong.com.

For information about special discounts for bulk purchases, please contact Simon & Schuster Special Sales at 1-866-506-1949 or business@simonandschuster.com.

The Simon & Schuster Speakers Bureau can bring authors to your live event. For more information or to book an event, contact the Simon & Schuster Speakers Bureau at 1-866-248-3049 or visit our website at www.simonspeakers.com.

Interior design by Priscilla Yuen
Interior images © Adobe Stock

Manufactured in the United States of America

1 2025

Library of Congress Control Number: 2025940321

ISBN 978-1-5072-2411-3
ISBN 978-1-5072-2412-0 (ebook)

Many of the designations used by manufacturers and sellers to distinguish their products are claimed as trademarks. Where those designations appear in this book and Simon & Schuster, LLC, was aware of a trademark claim, the designations have been printed with initial capital letters.

This book is intended as general information only and should not be used to diagnose or treat any health condition. Considering the complex, individual, and specific nature of health problems, this book is not intended to replace professional medical advice. You should always consult a trained medical professional before starting a diet, taking any form of medication, or embarking on any fitness or weight training program. The ideas, procedures, and suggestions in this book are intended to supplement, not replace, the advice of a trained medical professional. The author and publisher disclaim any liability arising directly or indirectly from the use of this book.

For Nonnie.
Without you, I wouldn't be me.

Contents

Contents | 5

CHAPTER 3 Nutrition Blueprint ... 71

CHAPTER 4 **Lifestyle Update** ... 137

CHAPTER 5 Transitioning Off GLP-1s ... 191

Introduction

In a world where information is all around you on social media channels or coming from your friends and family, it can be overwhelming to navigate a new medication in your health journey. What's right and what's wrong? How do you maximize your weight loss? How do you avoid side effects or manage those side effects that aren't avoidable? With numerous valid questions and a sea of misinformation, it's hard to know what's true and what's not. Fortunately, *The GLP-1 Solution* is here to help.

With this book, you'll find the answers to your most pressing questions about GLP-1s, starting right from the beginning where you'll find a chapter explaining all the basics of your new medication. Next, you'll discover more than 175 realistic strategies covering everything from side effects and nutrition to lifestyle changes and transitioning off your medication. Use these tips to help you feel empowered on your GLP-1 journey. Feel free to read the entries in order or flip through the pages until you find the one that you need in the moment.

Inside you'll uncover insights on:

- Your medication and how it's working in your body
- How to maximize your weight loss efforts
- How to avoid (or at least curb) side effects
- Handling dose increases and reductions
- Maintaining your weight loss once you stop your medication
- Lifestyle changes you can start right now to give yourself the best results possible!

Whether you are just now taking your first dose, are in the midst of your GLP-1 weight loss, or are weaning off the medication, think of this book as your solution to all your most pressing questions, concerns, and issues. These strategies, tips, and techniques are easy to follow, are easy to customize to suit your personal needs, and will help you feel confident every step of the way. Let's get started on a healthier you!

1

GLP-1 Basics

The world of GLP-1s can be overwhelming at first, especially when you realize how much information is out in the world about these medications. By the end of this chapter, you should feel more comfortable and confident in pursuing your GLP-1 journey. Any time you are prescribed a new medication, there's a good chance you'll have numerous questions, so let's start at the beginning with the basics. This chapter will explain how GLP-1s work in your body and how they help you lose weight, and provide an overview of the dieting and maintenance phases of being on these medications.

What Are GLP-1s?

Your body naturally produces the glucagon-like peptide-1 (GLP-1) hormone. One of the main roles of this hormone is to regulate your blood sugar, also known as glucose. Keeping your blood sugar balanced is necessary for weight loss. Your blood sugar level is largely determined by the foods you eat, but it can also be influenced by other lifestyle factors such as exercise, sleep, and stress.

When you have too much glucose in your bloodstream, your body continues to release more insulin—a hormone that tells your cells to soak up the glucose from the bloodstream into your cells. That rise in insulin signals the body to slow down on burning fat and instead store it in your fat cells. If this process repeats too often you develop a condition known as *insulin resistance*. When your body is insulin resistant it continuously makes and releases more insulin, which overwhelms your system, causing a host of problems and making weight loss much more challenging.

Conversely, if you were to have a drop in insulin levels your body would begin burning more fat. This is where the GLP-1 hormone comes in. This hormone improves insulin sensitivity and helps slow down digestion, which makes you feel fuller longer and less likely to eat in excess. However, the problem is that the GLP-1 hormone produced naturally by your body lasts only a very short time (often just a few minutes). This led scientists to try to create a synthetic version of the hormone that would mimic all the benefits of the natural hormone but would last longer for better results. And hence GLP-1 medications were born.

How GLP-1 Medications Work

Your natural GLP-1 hormone triggers your pancreas to release insulin, slows your gastric emptying (how quickly your stomach empties), makes you feel full after meals (satiety), and regulates glucagon secretion (a hormone that raises blood sugar). GLP-1 medications essentially do these same tasks in your body. GLP-1 medications attach to your cells and release a more potent and longer-lasting dose of GLP-1 than your body naturally does. These medications do not magically burn fat; they merely keep your blood sugar balanced to help you maintain a caloric deficit and therefore lose weight.

Slowing the Gastric Emptying Process and Improving Satiety

Gastric emptying is the speed at which food goes from your stomach to your small intestine. By slowing this gastric emptying with GLP-1 medications, you digest your food at a slower rate because it remains in your stomach longer than usual. This in turn helps regulate your insulin response, supports stable blood sugar levels, and makes you feel fuller faster. It's also likely that your portion sizes will need to be smaller because your stomach won't have the same capacity while you're on a GLP-1 medication.

Since you're digesting slower, this can help you feel full longer. This feeling of fullness and contentment after a meal is referred to as satiety; it's that feeling that you don't need more food because you have reached a satisfying fullness level. GLP-1 medications also influence the brain pathways that signal to your body that you are full, so they are working double time to provide support in this area. With slower gastric emptying and increased satiety, you will typically consume fewer calories, which can lead to weight loss.

Decreasing the Production of Glucagon

It's been shown through clinical studies that people with type 2 diabetes or those who struggle with obesity have higher levels of glucagon. GLP-1 medications help your body decrease the production of glucagon. With the help of GLP-1s, your glucagon secretion will moderate and be better able to work in sync with your insulin production. This creates a healthier blood sugar response, supports lower inflammation levels, and then can lead to potential weight loss.

Creating Stable Insulin Release

As mentioned earlier, the most important role of insulin in the context of GLP-1 medications is its role in managing blood sugar levels. If you have glucose (sugar) sitting in your bloodstream for too long, or have other issues related to insulin levels, you may have difficulty with weight loss. That's where your GLP-1 medication comes in; it creates a more effective and stable insulin response, which better controls your blood sugar levels and can help you prevent weight gain, or even lose weight.

Types of GLP-1 Medications

There are several kinds of GLP-1 medications on the market right now. These medications have various names including GLP-1 receptor agonists, GLP-1 agonists, and GIP (glucose-dependent insulinotropic polypeptide) receptor agonists. However, for the purposes of this book, we will refer to the entire class of these drugs as "GLP-1." The GLP-1 medications on the market all work in similar ways with slight variations, and they all have had slightly different results in their clinical trials and in real life.

Injectable GLP-1 medications include dulaglutide, exenatide, liraglutide, lixisenatide, and semaglutide. Semaglutide is one of the most commonly prescribed GLP-1s, sold under the brand names Ozempic and Wegovy. There's also an oral version called Rybelsus. Oral semaglutide can be a great option if you are needle averse, are prone to injection site reactions, travel a lot and can't keep your injections with you, or simply just prefer it. Your prescribing physician may also recommend one version over another for you specifically; it's important to discuss the options with your provider to determine which best fits your preference, wallet, and insurance coverage.

If you're taking tirzepatide, which is sold under the brand names Mounjaro or Zepbound, you may be wondering why it's not listed as a GLP-1 medication. Tirzepatide is a dual GLP-1 and GIP receptor agonist medication, so it's a slightly different drug; clinical trials have shown tirzepatide to have a bigger impact on weight loss than semaglutide.

The various GLP-1 medications mentioned here work similarly enough that outcomes are positive when it comes to improving your health. Their side effects are also very similar. In fact, no matter which one from among this class of medications that you're taking, the material in this book will be useful for you.

In closing, when looking at types of GLP-1 medications it is important to discuss the uncertainty and potential risks of compound versions. When commercial versions of a drug are difficult to obtain, often due to high demand, compounding pharmacies are allowed to make similar medications to fill the gap. However, these medications are not FDA-approved, and they don't go through the same rigorous safety and efficacy testing as brand-name drugs. And some vendors may use non-FDA-approved ingredients or operate in legal gray areas, putting patients at risk. Legitimate compounding pharmacies like 503A and 503B pharmacies do have standards for quality and safety. Consult a healthcare provider before considering a compounded version to ensure you're making a safe and informed decision.

Injection Information

If you have been prescribed an injectable medication, you may have some reservations about injecting yourself. You are not alone; this is often a new concept for many people. Fortunately, the process is fairly easy. When you pick up your medication, the pharmacy may include a chart that shows the possible injection sites; these usually include the stomach, the thighs, and the backs of the arms. These sites were chosen because they all allow you to inject into the fatty tissue right under your skin. This is important for GLP-1 medications because they are meant to be absorbed slowly over time; injecting into fatty tissue helps make that possible.

If you use your stomach as the injection site, you should stay at least two inches away from your belly button. To inject in your thigh, you'll want to use the top of the thigh toward the outside of your body. For your arm, use the back of the arm where you have the most fatty tissue. You should work with your medical provider to determine the best injection site and get a full list of injection instructions. As always, it's important to advocate for yourself if you'd prefer a different injection site than what your provider recommends.

When picking your injection site, to minimize the risk for injection site reactions, be sure to rotate your injection site. For thigh or arm injections, this can be rotating sides week to week; for abdominal injections you'll want to rotate around your abdomen each week. Everyone is unique and a particular injection site that works for one person might not be the right fit for another. It's important to find what's best for you when taking your medication.

Navigating Dose Increases

When taking any medication, knowledge is power, especially when there are several possible dose levels. GLP-1 medications typically start with the lowest dose possible, often called a loading dose. This low dose is taken for the first four weeks of your medication journey. From there, dose increases are driven by your progress, but also can be influenced by what your physician is used to.

It is important to note that you do not have to increase your dose if you are content with how the medicine is currently working. There could be a few different reasons for choosing not to up your dose: You may be happy with your current pace of weight loss, you may be happy with your lack of side effects, or, on the flip side, you may be struggling to tolerate side effects, or uncomfortable with seeing weight come off extremely fast. With dose increases, side effects typically increase. Common side effects of GLP-1 medications include fatigue, nausea, and constipation; this book offers many tips and techniques for how to deal with any side effects you may experience. Weight loss does usually happen faster at higher doses; however, if your metabolism isn't healthy, that won't be the case. Before increasing your GLP-1 dose, be sure to ask yourself if your side effects are well managed, if you are able to eat enough calories on your current dose, and if you desire to go up in dose.

Eventually most people will need to increase their dose due to natural plateaus. This is an appropriate response to the body adapting to its current stimuli and needing more medication to have the same effect. If your weight loss has plateaued or your lab work is not improving further (or is getting worse), a dose increase may be just the fix. There is, however, a cap for the highest dose you can take on GLP-1 medications, so there is a metaphorical ceiling. By leaving dose adjustments for when they are absolutely necessary, it allows you to extend your weight loss journey on GLP-1s for as long as possible. Ultimately, use caution, exercise your best judgment, and remember to advocate for yourself in any situation where medication adjustments are being discussed.

Phases of Nutrition on GLP-1s

While GLP-1 medications do support weight loss, it's important to stress that taking a GLP-1 does not guarantee that you will automatically lose weight. Weight loss is more complex and requires lifestyle modifications, nutrition changes, and a properly functioning metabolism to be paired with medication to see the best outcomes for your health. With the medication in your body setting you up for weight loss, it's up to you to follow through with healthy lifestyle and nutrition habits to achieve success. There are two phases of nutrition for people taking GLP-1 medications: the dieting phase, in which you will eat in a calorie deficit, and the maintenance phase, in which you will eat at your normal or maintenance calorie amount. During your GLP-1 journey, you will cycle between these two phases. Here is an explanation of these phases.

Dieting Phase

Weight loss isn't a guarantee, but pairing your GLP-1 medication with a dieting phase can help you progress toward the weight loss goal you've set for yourself. A dieting phase can be described as an intentional calorie deficit period during which you restrict a specific amount of daily calories to support weight loss. You will want to be in anywhere from a 15–20 percent calorie deficit from your maintenance calories as decided earlier by you and your healthcare provider. It's imperative that you avoid falling into the low-calorie and low-carbohydrate trap that is often set for you by society and social media; it will only come back to sabotage your progress in the future (you'll learn more about avoiding that later in this book).

The average person can accomplish 1–2 pounds of weight loss per week safely while at a 15–20 percent calorie deficit. On average, human bodies will respond to dieting phases for around twelve months maximum, but that's only if you are doing a safe and sustainable calorie deficit (no fad diets or crash diets). With the combination of a GLP-1 medication and a calorie deficit, you may see a larger initial drop on the scale that will then slow to a less rapid, sustainable pace over time. This is typically attributed to an initial decrease in inflammation and then the loss of fat follows.

One of the biggest challenges people experience with weight loss is keeping the weight off in the long run. An almost guaranteed way to eventually gain all the weight back is to eat too few calories or not enough carbohydrates, or stay in a dieting period too long. You cannot remain in a dieting phase indefinitely; your body is not meant to be on a diet forever. After your dieting phase, you must spend time eating enough during your maintenance phase.

Maintenance Phase

To be able to sustain your weight loss long term, it's important to take care of your metabolism. Even with a GLP-1 medication on board, you cannot ignore or outrun your metabolism. Your metabolism is your body's survival mechanism. Your body cannot differentiate as to why you are choosing to restrict food intake; it just knows there is less food, so your metabolism adapts, slowing down to adjust to your food intake. Adding food back in small, frequent amounts from your deficit calories up to your maintenance calories will allow you to maintain a healthy metabolism and give your body a break.

Whether you have lost all the weight you were hoping to lose or are simply needing to give your body a break from dieting, maintenance phases are key to lasting results. A maintenance phase is intentional time spent eating at your maintenance calories, no calorie deficit in sight, and also not eating in a surplus (which can cause weight gain). Your body functions at its optimal health when it is being properly nourished, and that's at maintenance.

Depending on the amount of weight loss you are aiming for, you may need to cycle through several rounds of maintenance phases and calorie deficits to be able to reach your final weight loss goal safely and sustainably.

Your GLP-1 Journey Is Yours

As a final thought to wrap up the basics, please know that your GLP-1 journey is yours and yours alone. Everyone has an opinion about everything these days, and GLP-1 medications are no different. They can often come with stigma, so if you have made the decision to take a GLP-1 medication (or if you are contemplating making that choice), try to ignore the naysayers and focus on what's really important: your health. With the help of this book, you should feel empowered to make the most informed health decision for you. Utilize this new knowledge to guide you to the healthiest version of yourself.

2 | Side Effect Roadmap

One of the main reasons someone would stop taking their GLP-1 medication is because they are having unmanageable side effects. Nausea, vomiting, constipation, diarrhea, fatigue, and even hair loss can be common occurrences when taking a GLP-1 medication. These side effects are typically experienced most when your lifestyle isn't in check. It's often just a simple lack of awareness that leads some people to discontinue their GLP-1 medication and lose out on the life-changing experience they could've had.

Thankfully, almost every side effect that comes with GLP-1 medications can be managed to the point where it's barely noticeable or eliminated completely; this requires the knowledge of why the issue happens and the tools to battle it. In this chapter, you will learn how to navigate the bumpy road that can come with side effects from GLP-1 medications. You will not only learn how to combat the side effects in the moment, but you will also learn how to prevent them from occurring in the first place.

You will be able to have a successful and healthy experience on your GLP-1 medication with these practical applications to keep you side effect–free.

1   Navigating Nausea

Nausea is one of the most reported side effects from GLP-1 medications and it's also one of the easiest to navigate with the right tools. When you are nauseated, accomplishing even the simplest task can become a monumental feat. When you think of nausea, you may think of your stomach feeling unsettled, feeling like you might vomit, or an uneasy feeling in your throat, but it can also feel like a loss of appetite, dizziness, and excess sweating.

You may notice that when you first start your GLP-1 medication your nausea is at its worst. This can be very common and should typically subside within four to eight weeks for most people. The second most common time you can experience nausea on your GLP-1 is if you have an increase in your medication dose. A quick rule is that the higher the dose you have, the worse the nausea typically is.

Two tools to battle nausea that don't require you to buy anything or go anywhere are controlled breathing and staying rested.

- You can practice controlled breathing by focusing on a 4-second breath in and a 4-second breath out over several minutes to help settle any nauseated feelings.
- Resting enough throughout the day and getting enough sleep at night have been shown to support digestion and help lower nausea levels. The saying "rest is best" is especially important in terms of battling nausea.

2 | Shrink Your Meals

A major change that comes with taking your GLP-1 medication is a reduction in your portion sizes. If you are someone who is used to eating larger meals only once or twice a day, your meal size will need to change if you want to minimize your side effects.

Because your digestion slows down on GLP-1 medications, you will need to reduce your portion sizes so that you can walk away from your meals without being stuffed full or feeling sick. When you overeat at meals while taking a GLP-1, you are going to experience a prolonged sense of discomfort and fullness. If you have food that has been sitting for too long in your stomach, your body will find a way to get that food out. This usually results in either vomiting or diarrhea.

In addition to your overall meal size decreasing, you will also want to be mindful of your specific serving sizes of proteins, carbohydrates, and fats. Protein should be your top priority at meals with fats being secondary and carbohydrates last. If you are struggling with fullness, post-meal illness, nausea, or indigestion, do a quick evaluation of your actual meal composition to see if you need to reduce those specific ratios to create a more balanced meal.

3 | Increase Your Meal Frequency

With the need to decrease your meal sizes into smaller portions, you'll need to create more meal opportunities throughout the day. When taking GLP-1 medications, constipation, low blood sugar, and undereating can all appear as side effects as you are adjusting to a new normal. If you can keep the thought of small, frequent meals in your mind throughout the day, you'll be setting yourself up to be side effect–free.

In terms of digestion, one of the best things you can do to support regular breakdown of food and regular bowel movements is to have regular meals throughout the day. Another way to help avoid constipation is to be sure you are consuming enough food overall; if you aren't eating enough, there's not going to be much to be digested!

Enjoying well-balanced meals throughout the day is also important as that allows you to maintain a more stable blood sugar level and avoid low blood sugar episodes. If you are going prolonged periods without eating, it can create dips in your blood sugar levels that will leave you feeling shaky and nauseated. Small, frequent meals can help with this.

Finally, as your portion sizes have decreased to accommodate for slower digestion, your calories per meal have also decreased. Therefore, if you don't increase your meal frequency, you'll end up undereating, which will cause a host of side effects you'll want to avoid. Creating a regular meal schedule that spans throughout the whole day will help you get all the calories you need, while also supporting your blood sugar levels and avoiding constipation.

4   Create a Bland Food Buffer

Whether your indigestion is being triggered by the slower digestion from your GLP-1, your food choices, or other lifestyle habits you haven't solidified yet to make life easier on your medication, adding in bland food can help alleviate indigestion quickly. Typically, alcohol, caffeine, citrus, spicy foods, and carbonation can all worsen indigestion and are best to limit where you can. Bland foods can help create a buffer during meals and bring your indigestion down so it's not unbearable.

Often when people think of bland foods, they think of bananas, rice, applesauce, and toast. And while these foods are all technically bland, they lack major nutrients like protein that are important for you to keep in all your meals while taking GLP-1 medications. You should aim to include a wider variety of bland foods to stay nourished and have relief from indigestion.

For proteins, leaner meats like chicken or ground turkey, eggs, plain low-fat yogurt, and bone broth can all be good additions to a bland diet. In terms of fruit, in addition to applesauce and bananas you can try melon or canned fruits without added sugars. Along with the usual rice, you can also add in bread, pastas, and crackers, ideally from white flour to make them easier to digest in the short term. Rounding out your plate, for vegetables avoid cruciferous vegetables like broccoli or Brussels sprouts and aim to include fully cooked vegetables like carrots, peas, beets, or spinach.

5 | Pace Yourself While Eating

The pace at which you eat can have major impacts on your ability to digest your food well. If rushing through your meals sounds familiar, you may also relate to the bloating, indigestion, and discomfort that typically follows those meals. Even if you are used to a quicker-paced meal without any indigestion or bloating, you may start to experience these symptoms while taking your GLP-1 medication.

When you eat too quickly, you take in more air with each swallow, which will lead to increased bloating. Typically, when you are rushing a meal you also are chewing it less, which means your food isn't broken down as much as it should be by the time it hits your stomach and you're going to experience more heartburn plus bloating. Thankfully, there is a fix that you can implement for quick relief.

While you are enjoying your meals, you want to slow the entire process down from start to finish. This starts with a calm eating environment so you can focus on slowing down and savoring your food. You should try to put your utensils down in between bites so you can chew thoroughly, swallow, and take a few breaths before your next bite. Be sure to also keep your mealtimes regular throughout the day so you don't go too long without eating. If you do have to be on the move while eating, try to take a few full breaths in between bites to avoid eating your food too quickly. If you've always had quicker mealtimes, give yourself time to adjust to this new, slower pace.

6 Chew Thoroughly for Relief

A major component of digestion isn't something your body does automatically. It is unfortunately also something that a lot of people cut short, which can lead to more frequent indigestion and bloating. This illusive component of digestion is . . . chewing!

It may seem obvious to say that you have to chew your food before swallowing, but more often than not when someone is struggling with indigestion and bloating, it can be linked back to not chewing properly and starting the digestion process off on the wrong foot. When you don't chew your food thoroughly, you send food into your stomach in bigger pieces. This then requires more work from your digestive enzymes and stomach acid to break the food down into small enough pieces to move into the small intestine for nutrient absorption. While your stomach is working harder to digest the food, that food sits longer in your stomach and can create uncomfortable bloating and abdominal distention paired with indigestion.

To alleviate this problem, you first want to create an environment for your meals that's free of distractions (like screens) and that's ideally not on the go. If you can't avoid eating on the go, try to remove other distractions to focus on chewing. You could try counting in your head up to ten, twenty, or even thirty chews before swallowing, or you can try to bring awareness to each bite and ensure you take the time to chew for several seconds before each swallow. If you can train yourself to chew more and slow down while eating, it'll help keep the indigestion and bloating at bay.

7   Avoid Strong Scents

While smelling something you dislike can normally cause nausea, when this experience is combined with taking a GLP-1 medication it can be an unwelcome double whammy. For some people, only very strong scents like gasoline, cigarettes, or cleaning products can create an adverse reaction; however, what triggers you is completely individual. Perfumes, nail polishes, or even certain foods like fish can all elicit strong scent aversions that can create a gagging sensation or simply increase your nausea levels, leading to discomfort.

A good rule is to steer clear of strong scents you know typically irritate you if you are already battling nausea from your GLP-1 medication. However, this isn't always possible and sometimes you can even find yourself experiencing nausea from a scent that doesn't normally bother you. So what can you do? A quick tip would be to keep Vicks VapoRub or Aquaphor Healing Ointment with you so if you encounter an unpleasant smell you can create a buffer by covering the offensive smell with the strong scent of these products. Just remember that a little goes a long way! You can also keep peppermints handy to suck on, carry small first-aid alcohol swabs with you (smelling these can help alleviate nausea), or even wear a mask to help filter out some of the smell.

8 | Change Your Injection Time

The timing of your injection is truly up to you. But it's important to remember that the timing of your shot can be moved around to best accommodate not only your schedule but also your side effects.

For some people, the timing of their weekly injection doesn't make a big impact on side effects, but for others controlling the timing can make a big difference overall. Changing the timing of your injection can help mitigate side effects like fatigue or nausea. One simple swap can make a significant dent in how you are feeling post injection. Here are some helpful solutions:

- If you are someone who struggles with fatigue after your shot, doing your injection on a weekday can make it difficult to make it through those following workdays without taking a nap to battle the fatigue. Instead, try swapping your injection to the day before you have your weekend (like Fridays) so you can take some extra rest time and return to work after the fatigue has worn off.

- If you are someone who experiences nausea after your injection, consider swapping your injection time to right before bed. This will allow you to sleep through the first few hours and it can help offset some of the initial onset of nausea. For some, the nausea right after the injection isn't even a product of the medication itself but rather from the actual process of injecting. Sleeping through this time can help mitigate this feeling.

Finding the injection time that works best for you and your body will make a huge difference in how you feel physically and mentally.

9 Get to Know Ginger

Ginger is about to be your new best friend, and while it's not a magic cure, it does have anti-nausea properties that can help you feel better. Since your GLP-1 medication slows down digestion, food is sitting in your stomach longer than it normally used to. When food remains in your stomach too long, it can create worsening nausea and make you feel miserable. Rather than taking a nausea medication that can cause constipation, try ginger instead.

The gingerol compound in gingerroot supports motility in your gastrointestinal tract, aka your gut. So, when you consume ginger, it can help support the stomach emptying and create relief from the nausea.

Ginger can be consumed in multiple ways including:

- Store-bought ginger teas
- Hard ginger candies or chews
- Ginger paste
- Crystalized ginger (It's important to note that this does have a higher sugar count; if you are watching your sugar intake, a different option may be best for you.)
- Ginger supplements (Be sure to select your supplement from a company that utilizes third-party testing so you know it's a safe option for you.)

If you're up for a little DIY, you can buy fresh gingerroot from the store, peel it at home, and combine with boiling water to create your own ginger tea.

10 Utilize the Benefits of Chamomile

If you are struggling with indigestion or an upset stomach, chamomile tea should be in your rotation. Chamomile tea is an easy and effective choice as it is generally well tolerated by most people, comes with a low price tag, and can be found at almost every grocery store or online retailer.

Chamomile tea is packed with antioxidants that can have a soothing effect on the digestive tract. So, while a cup of chamomile tea doesn't directly lower indigestion and reflux, it does calm the inflammation that indigestion can cause. When inflammation is soothed, it can create symptom relief and make your digestive issues more tolerable and easier to resolve with other lifestyle modifications.

To utilize chamomile tea, grab tea bags at your local grocery store and then steep one tea bag for 5–10 minutes in 8–10 ounces of hot water. Sip it slowly to avoid liquid overload, which can lead to abdominal discomfort. Of course, for the best results follow the instructions of the specific brand of tea you buy.

Despite the tea's many benefits, there are some groups of people who should steer clear of chamomile tea; these include anyone with a ragweed allergy and folks on blood-thinning medications. You should consult your physician if you feel you might have an issue with trying chamomile teas.

11 | Stay Upright

While lying down and resting is always encouraged, the one time it's discouraged is after your meals, especially if you are struggling with indigestion, reflux, bloating, and nausea. In fact, one of the worst things you can do if you want to alleviate your reflux is lie down.

When you lie down, especially when your stomach is full right after a meal, it is easier for your stomach acid to roll back up into your esophagus, which will end up with you having to add in more interventions to bring down the reflux so you can get comfortable. Instead of having to try more interventions, you can focus on staying upright and skip the post-meal reflux altogether.

The first way to avoid this problem is simple, just stay upright! Stand or sit; as long as your upper body is upright, your digestive system can work its magic. While on a GLP-1, many people find that they need to stay upright for longer periods of time after a meal than before they started their medication. This tends to be around 60 minutes for most people, but pay attention to how you feel to find your own individual time. The second way does require a bit more effort, but you can easily stay upright for a period of time by walking around. You can walk in your house, on a treadmill, or even outside; it doesn't matter where, as long as you're on the move! You get a few bonus steps in, stay upright, and as a final bonus, walking after meals can actually help stabilize your blood sugar and move your digestion along.

12 Wear Loose-Fitting Clothes

It may seem unconventional to be told to loosen up your clothes, especially in today's world where most of the fashion choices lean toward tighter clothing. Whether that tightness comes from the natural compression of athletic wear, from a personal preference for tighter-fitting styles, or from not having properly fitting clothes at the moment, clothes that are too tight can actually affect your digestion. As wild as it may sound, tight clothing can make your indigestion, bloating, and even nausea worse.

From a digestion standpoint, tight clothing like jeans, belts, compressive athletic wear, or compression undergarments can create indigestion or worsen reflux issues. The pressure that the clothing puts on your stomach can cause your stomach acid to push back up through the esophageal sphincter. The same tight garments can also restrict normal gas movement through your gastrointestinal tract, which can lead to abdominal pain and bloating. When both bloating and indigestion increase, your nausea levels can also increase as a result. Tight garments around your neck like turtlenecks can also put pressure on your throat, which can worsen any nausea you may be experiencing.

So, although it may sound odd for a healthcare provider to tell you to loosen up your clothes, it can make a major difference in how you feel. Try swapping out your compressive athletic wear for looser options, size up if you're able to grab some new clothing items, tuck the turtlenecks away, and leave the belt at home.

13 Cool Your Body Down

Embracing the cold isn't for everyone, but it can be one of the quickest ways to alleviate nausea. Even in extreme situations where you may be feeling close to vomiting, cooling your body down can help you avoid becoming physically ill and can even go as far as alleviating the nausea altogether.

When your body is feeling nauseated, typically you experience a rise in body temperature. How warm you get does vary depending on your individual body and your environment, but that increase in body temperature and warmth in the surrounding environment can increase nausea and induce vomiting if it escalates far enough. You can knock out the nausea, however, by quickly cooling down your body.

If the weather is cooperative and it's chilly outside, getting out into the fresh, chill air for several minutes can help nausea wind down and relax your body. If there's not a cold weather opportunity, you can simulate one with air-conditioning. Crank up the air-conditioning unit in your home or car as much as possible and station your body right next to those air vents for a quick cool down. You can also use cold compresses and ice packs. Place the coldest compress you can find on your head, back of your neck, or chest to help with symptom relief. Any other areas of your body that are feeling unreasonably warm can also be targeted with a cold compress. By keeping these cold compresses on rotation you can keep your body temperature lower and hopefully escape the nausea.

14 Use Peppermint

Peppermint can save you from most of your GLP-1–related digestion side effects. Constipation, reflux, and nausea can all be improved with a bit of peppermint. Peppermint, which contains anti-inflammatory ingredients like menthol, helps by relaxing the smooth muscles in your digestive system and soothing any involuntary muscle spasms. The beauty of peppermint is that there are multiple ways you can implement it.

Two popular options are peppermint teas and peppermint capsules. Peppermint teas are easy to grab at your local grocery store or online retailer and usually have a reasonable price point. Peppermint teas tend to be best for nausea or reflux. Peppermint capsules are a great option to keep in your medicine cabinet and can be found easiest in online retailers. These capsules are most effective in alleviating constipation.

Peppermint oil can additionally be helpful in topical form for addressing gastrointestinal symptoms; however, it can take several days to weeks to be effective so it's not the quickest course of action. No matter which method you choose, stock up on your peppermint products so when symptoms strike, you're ready for battle.

15 Choose the Appropriate Constipation Remedy

When taking GLP-1 medications, almost everyone will experience constipation at some point; however, the degree to which you are constipated will vary. Ideally, you will want to implement natural remedies before resorting to laxatives, but laxatives can be beneficial when paired with medical supervision to prevent further complications from constipation. Let's compare the main points and benefits of each so you can make the choice that is best for you and your situation.

Natural remedies range from habits, to supplements, to specific foods. For example, habits to address constipation can include massage, acupuncture, or stretching. Supplements can include fiber powders, probiotics, flaxseed, or magnesium. Foods can include kiwis or prunes. All these natural remedies aim to promote bowel movements and alleviate constipation through movement, softening stools, and stimulating the colon without medication interventions. These methods can be helpful for preventing severe constipation but may not be enough alone if your constipation becomes too severe.

Over-the-counter laxatives primarily aim to soften the stool, to add bulk to stool to make bowel movements easier to pass, or to stimulate a bowel movement. Most laxatives can be purchased over the counter but should be used with caution as they can cause dehydration. Laxatives are typically used to alleviate constipation that's more acute to avoid developing bowel blockages.

16   Find Relief with Magnesium Citrate

There are several different forms of magnesium on the market. While you'd want magnesium glycinate for overall health, magnesium citrate should be your choice when dealing with constipation.

If your constipation is approaching the point of needing laxative intervention, but you'd like to put off using the big gun laxatives, you should try magnesium citrate. It's considered to be a more natural laxative option. You can find it in capsule form or liquid form; however, most people report a more gentle effect with the capsule form. Magnesium citrate works by increasing water in the small intestine to help soften and move your stool out of you. As long as you don't take too much at once, it can be a very mild but effective intervention. For most people, anywhere from 250–420 milligrams per day can result in a bowel movement but be sure to read the instructions on the product you buy.

Keep in mind, magnesium citrate is not a long-term solution for constipation and shouldn't be overused. It can be a great tool on occasion, but you'll want to ensure that you are able to pass the majority of your bowel movements without magnesium citrate.

Bonus tip if you find you get extra constipated while traveling since starting your GLP-1: Add in magnesium citrate at a low dose before leaving for your trip and for a few days after travel to help keep the bowels moving!

17 Try Kiwis for Constipation

What if you could alleviate your constipation with just two kiwis per day? It's a fairly simple addition to your day that could give you major relief from constipation. The great news is that science says that two kiwis a day can indeed relieve constipation and support regular bowel movements.

You will need to take into account that most kiwis you can find at your local grocery store will need a few days to soften up before they're ready to eat, so you likely will want to keep kiwi on your grocery list to grab a few each time you head to the store. Additionally, the relief from kiwi requires several days to take effect for most people; however, once you have them in your daily fruit intake, a two-a-day kiwi habit should provide constipation relief.

Kiwis are thought to relieve your constipation as a result of their soluble and insoluble fiber content, water content, and a digestive enzyme they contain called actinidin. Fiber and water content help soften stool and pull water into your colon to help bowel movements pass. Actinidin supports your gastric emptying and can stimulate receptors that are found in your colon. The saying that food can be medicine couldn't be truer where kiwi is involved.

18 Experiment with Prunes for Irregularity

Mild to moderate constipation can be resolved and even prevented with regular prune intake. Incorporating prunes into your diet on a daily basis, over multiple days to weeks, can create a natural solution for the constipation that can come as a side effect of your GLP-1 medication.

Prunes carry a few key properties that can make them helpers for avoiding major constipation episodes. They contain water-soluble fiber, polyphenols, and sorbitol, all of which contribute to producing a bowel movement. The fiber and sorbitol are important for pulling water into the intestines to keep stool soft and moving. Polyphenols also help regulate bowel movements.

Even if prunes aren't your favorite-tasting food, as a relatively low-risk intervention to keep constipation away or resolve constipation, their benefits can certainly outweigh their shortcomings. The serving size of prunes that has been shown to help alleviate constipation is only 100 grams per day. Prune juice can also help with some cases of constipation; however, there's no established recommendation for what amount to drink, so you will have to experiment with how much you need to drink daily to alleviate or prevent constipation.

If the taste of prunes is not to your liking, you can try to mask the taste by adding a small (dime-sized) dollop of nut butter on each prune. If you're experimenting with prune juice instead, try incorporating it into a mixed berry smoothie to improve the taste!

19 | Look Into Laxatives

Laxatives can be over the counter or prescribed by your physician. They're primarily used to treat constipation in a variety of settings. Whether the constipation is travel induced, lifestyle induced, occurring after surgeries, or a side effect of a medication like GLP-1s, laxatives help keep your bowels moving so you don't end up with serious complications as a result of constipation. Remaining constipated for long periods of time can cause nausea, vomiting, hemorrhoids, anal fissures, and even impactions and blockages in your intestines. All of these results are extremely uncomfortable and take a considerable amount of further medical attention and care to solve. Thankfully, laxatives can help you avoid all the complications that can come from being constipated.

There are three main types of laxatives: stimulant laxatives, osmotic laxatives, and bulk laxatives (see the next entry for more on bulk laxatives). Stimulant laxatives work by stimulating the muscles and nerves in your colon to produce a bowel movement. Osmotic laxatives work by pulling water from your body into your intestines to soften the stool and make it easier to pass. The specifics of your constipation situation will determine which type of laxative is best for you. Stimulant laxatives typically lead to a bowel movement within several hours, while osmotic laxatives produce a bowel movement within a few days.

If you are experiencing constipation to the point where you are wondering if you need a laxative, either over the counter or prescribed, you should consult your healthcare provider so they can help you make the most informed choice.

20 Stay Hydrated on Bulk-Forming Laxatives

Bulk-forming laxatives aren't your typical laxatives but they can be helpful for those taking GLP-1s because they help add substance to your bowel movements. This type of laxative works by increasing the weight of the stool that's forming in your intestines as well as by pulling water into the stool to keep it soft. This is a slower-acting laxative that takes several days to be fully effective, so it should not be used to try to produce a bowel movement quickly or if you are already severely constipated.

Since a bulk-forming laxative pulls water in and holds water to soften and create more weight in the stool, it can quickly lead to dehydration if you aren't staying on top of water intake while taking the laxative. Most laxatives in this category will instruct you to drink a full glass of water with the laxative itself. However, it is often better to drink at least half your body weight in ounces each day as a minimum to stay hydrated.

Bulk-forming laxatives also contain more fiber than other types of laxatives and can be a helpful tool as you are first adjusting to your new dietary intake on your GLP-1. Undereating in general is a common occurrence for many people taking GLP-1 medications. If you are coming up short with intake of fiber-rich foods such as fruits, vegetables, and whole grains, short-term use of a bulk-forming laxative can be helpful to boost fiber intake and support regular bowel movements.

Common bulk-forming laxatives include psyllium (Metamucil) and methylcellulose (Citrucel).

21 | Use Osmotic Laxatives with Caution

As a first-line option for constipation that's worsening, osmotic laxatives are commonly recommended and used to alleviate constipation. Typical turnaround time for osmotic laxatives to work for most people (this can vary depending on your constipation level, dose of your GLP-1, and your body) is two to three days.

Easily accessible at most local stores and online retailers, osmotic laxatives are most helpful for early stages of constipation. If you are using an osmotic laxative for more than a few days with no bowel movement produced, you'll want to consult your healthcare provider for next steps so your constipation does not worsen. Osmotic laxatives, like all laxatives, are a tool to be used occasionally; you should be able to manage any constipation most of the time with lifestyle changes only. The most common times to need a laxative while on a GLP-1 would be when first starting the medication, any time you increase your dose, or when making major dietary changes.

Since osmotic laxatives are pulling water into the intestines to create bowel movements, they can have side effects. If there's too much movement in your bowels, you can end up with diarrhea instead of a normal bowel movement. Osmotic laxatives also can lead to dehydration and electrolyte imbalances. If you are battling dehydration and having several bowel movements (formed or loose) in a short amount of time, it can cause your electrolytes to be thrown off balance. Symptoms of electrolyte imbalances can include lightheadedness, dizziness, excessive thirst, or confusion. If any of these occur for you, contact your healthcare provider immediately for support.

Common osmotic laxatives include Miralax, Glycolax, and Milk of Magnesia.

22 | Try Stool Softeners As a First Defense

While it is true that category-wise, stool softeners are still considered laxatives, they do differ in purpose. A primary reason to take a laxative is to produce a bowel movement in order to alleviate constipation. Stool softeners differ in that they do not *cause* a bowel movement to happen. Instead, stool softeners create wetter and softer stools to make them easier to pass when a bowel movement does happen. In the whole universe of laxatives, since stool softeners don't cause a bowel movement to happen, they're usually on the lower end of effectiveness for chronic constipation or severe constipation.

If the constipation that you're experiencing is related primarily to dehydration, a stool softener could help solve your problem. Stool softeners commonly are found in liquid form or enema form. If you decide to go the enema route, consult your physician for instructions.

Your ability to be in tune with your body and pinpoint what could be causing your constipation will help you decide if a stool softener would be an appropriate choice as a first-line defense before your constipation progresses. More often than not, early detection of oncoming constipation can be solved with a stool softener, extra water, and a little movement.

Common stool softeners include Colace and Correctol.

23 Get Quick Relief with Stimulant Laxatives

As one of the fastest-acting laxatives, stimulants can be an option for quicker constipation relief. Within 6–12 hours there's typically a bowel movement to provide relief. When the muscles and nerves in your colon are being stimulated, the contractions of the muscle increase, which physically pushes the stool out of you. Stool also typically can be softened with stimulant laxatives, making it easier to pass the bowel movement.

The most common forms of stimulant laxatives are suppositories and oral medications. Suppositories are small, usually round, medications that are inserted in the rectum to create the stimulant effect. If you choose to utilize a suppository, be sure to follow all instructions for the specific type you are using. Oral versions of stimulant laxatives can be found in liquid or capsule form as well. Your personal preference can lead the way to which type of laxative to try.

To have the most positive experience with stimulant laxatives, here are some best practices:

- Take the laxative at nighttime to ideally have a bowel movement in the morning.
- If you take the laxative during the day, be near enough to a bathroom in case you need to quickly get there.
- Increase your water intake to offset any potential dehydration.
- Use them sparingly and only when absolutely necessary.

Stimulant laxatives can lead to dependency and create long-term impacts on your bowel movements and bowel habits, so it's important to consult with your healthcare provider if you are needing to use them frequently; you might need to find a different solution.

Stimulant laxatives include Dulcolax and Senna.

24 Dealing with Diarrhea

An unfortunate side effect for some people taking GLP-1 medications is that diarrhea can be a common occurrence. This diarrhea isn't a result of trying to fix constipation or from overconsuming at mealtimes, though that is possible (more to come later on this), rather this diarrhea is a stand-alone side effect from the medication itself. For some people taking GLP-1 medications, the delayed gastric emptying that happens can cause diarrhea instead of constipation.

If diarrhea is affecting you, it typically will be at its worst when you first start your GLP-1 medication or after any dose increases. After one to four weeks, it should subside overall as a side effect for almost everyone. In the meantime, how can you manage diarrhea so it doesn't impact your daily life as much?

While your body is adjusting to your medication, you may need to maintain a blander diet to aid in easier digestion. It's not a forever change, just a temporary fix. If you are experiencing diarrhea, it's best to not skip meals as a way of trying to avoid a diarrhea episode. Instead, focus on smaller, frequent meals to help your digestive system have less work at a time. To build your diarrhea survival kit, see the upcoming Build a Diarrhea Toolkit entry to create your emergency plan if diarrhea strikes.

25 | Implement the BRAT Diet

The BRAT diet is a very specific way of eating that comes with a set of regulations to follow. It may not work for everyone, but it's something that you can try if diarrhea, nausea, or indigestion are bothering you. While the BRAT diet creates a bland diet, it is more restrictive than sticking to a wider variety of bland foods. The BRAT diet is intended for short-term use, typically during short periods of illness. This is not a recommended long-term solution for managing symptoms that are arising from taking a GLP-1 medication because it lacks protein, fiber, and a variety of nutrients.

If you find yourself actively ill with vomiting or diarrhea, your first step can be to implement the BRAT principles. BRAT stands for bananas, rice, applesauce, and toast. The fiber content will help solidify any loose stools and all four items are easy to digest to aid with any discomfort you may experience when you are sick. Traditionally, you will want to avoid any foods outside these four until you are free from illness. As you start to feel better, you can expand your food repertoire slowly back to normal. For most people, if they have been extremely sick, their stomachs can still be sensitive; if that's your experience, focus on adding in more variety. For ideas, flip back to the Create a Bland Food Buffer entry earlier in this chapter to get some ideas on options for creating balanced meals as you recover.

26 Build a Diarrhea Toolkit

If you find yourself in the unfortunate situation where diarrhea is becoming an everyday occurrence, you're going to want to be prepared and have an action plan. Some quick actions you can take to slow down diarrhea include:

- Focus on bland foods that are more carbohydrate heavy like breads, pastas, and rice.
- Avoid stimulants like caffeine and other irritants such as spicy foods, fatty foods, and carbonated beverages.
- Use over-the-counter medications like Imodium and Pepto Bismol for short-term relief.
- Take regular trips to the bathroom to avoid potential emergencies.
- Stay hydrated with water and consider adding electrolytes if you don't normally take them.
- Keep a small bag of medicine with you wherever you go, so if you happen to be out and about, you can get quick relief if diarrhea shows up.

In addition to being prepared to take quick action, it's important to be able to figure out why diarrhea is happening in the first place. If you're able to pinpoint that you took too many laxatives, pull back on your usage immediately to let your bowel movements regulate back to normal. If overeating at meals was the cause, try regulating your portion sizes in the future to help prevent you from suffering again.

27 | Evade Vomiting

Unfortunately, vomiting is a relatively common side effect with GLP-1 medications. To be able to evade vomiting, try this two-step process.

Step one involves understanding which of your habits may be predisposing you to a higher chance of experiencing vomiting. If you can check off any of the following, it's time for change:

- [ ] *You are eating large meals that leave you feeling uncomfortably full.*
- [ ] *Your meals are sporadically occurring throughout the day with no rhyme or reason.*
- [ ] *Your meals are high in fat or sugar or contain extra spicy foods.*
- [ ] *You're skimping on your water intake and are regularly dehydrated.*
- [ ] *You're consuming alcohol on a regular basis.*

All of the previous items can increase your chances of triggering vomiting when paired with taking a GLP-1 medication. Since you are aware now of areas of possible improvement, you can move to step two of your anti-vomiting strategy.

Step two has two parts: The first is to create a game plan to avoid any habits that may be triggers that predispose you to vomiting. The second part is to deter any active vomiting, whether it's already happening or you feel like it's about to happen. One of the best things you can do in this situation is to rest in a fully seated position, or in a propped-up position if you plan to lie down. You can also get some fresh air or try to distract yourself with your favorite movie, book, or podcast to avoid thinking about vomiting. As a last resort, you can work with your healthcare provider to get prescription nausea relief like Zofran to take if things escalate and no lifestyle interventions are helping.

28 | Use Ginseng for Fatigue

As your body is adjusting to being on a GLP-1 medication, fatigue can set in and make it hard to get through the day. In a perfect world, you'd have no fatigue or be able to consume unlimited caffeine to combat your fatigue. However, in the real world, the fatigue is real and unlimited caffeine will lead to you being jittery, having stomach issues, and overall not helping you to be productive. There is a solution, though, that does not involve bottomless cups of coffee. Instead of caffeine, you can incorporate ginseng to help offset the fatigue you're experiencing.

In terms of ginseng, you'll want to look for Asian ginseng, known as *Panax ginseng*, because this is the type of ginseng that's going to give you an energy boost. (American ginseng, known as *Panax quinquefolius*, is actually a calming agent, so it's best to avoid it if you're already tired.) In supplement form, it's believed that ginseng can help you at the cellular level by reducing oxidative stress. When your oxidative stress decreases, you see a reported increase in energy levels.

You can commonly find ginseng in over-the-counter supplements in capsule form. As for dose, studies have shown that 2,000–3,000 milligrams per day can improve fatigue levels. For anyone with an autoimmune disease or bipolar disorder, ginseng may be contraindicated. As always, consult with your healthcare provider to make sure it's safe for you to implement ginseng in your routine if you are feeling tired and want a boost.

29 Try the Pinch and Poke Test for Bloating

Chances are when you are evaluating your body to see if you're bloated while taking a GLP-1 medication, you might mistake bloating for fullness and normal distention. After you eat the first meal of the day, you will naturally start expanding. After a full day of eating, you will physically appear larger than you did in the morning and that can be seen primarily in your abdomen, which will protrude out more. Add in a GLP-1 medication that slows down your digestion, and chances are you will experience more distention than you did before taking the medication, since food is sitting in your stomach longer. Simply the presence of a fuller stomach and some additional protrusion, however, doesn't equate to bloating.

Bloating is a common symptom with GLP-1 medications and can be extremely uncomfortable. With bloating, there will also be distention; however, this distention typically includes pain, tightness, and a full feeling. It can also be accompanied by increased abdominal cramping and gas.

A quick test is the pinch and poke test. If you're bloated when you pinch your abdomen, it will likely result in discomfort or pain and be hard to fully pinch. And when you poke your abdomen, your finger will be met with more resistance. If you are just normally expanding from the meals and fluids throughout the day, it'll likely be a softer poke and you should be able to pinch up your abdominal skin without discomfort. This test isn't the be-all and end-all; if you suspect you're dealing with bloating and not normal fluctuations from food and drinks, notify your healthcare provider.

30 Beat the Bloat

The chance you have ended up bloated and uncomfortable on at least one occasion since starting your GLP-1 medication is almost guaranteed. It's an unfortunate side effect of GLP-1 medications. However, you do not have to be a prisoner to bloating; you can fight back and beat the bloat. Here are a few tips to tackle bloating:

- Identify any triggers like carbonated beverages and minimize them or avoid them altogether.
- Have smaller and more frequent meals throughout the day.
- Create a calm, distraction-free environment for your meals and snacks.
- Drink plenty of water to avoid dehydration.
- Go for a 5- to 10-minute walk after your main meals.
- Massage your abdomen in a U shape.
- Focus on stretching and mobility.

Without adding in any supplements, prescriptions, or additional foods, you can create significant improvements with bloating. The most underrated tip on this list is walking after meals. You don't even need to get outside; just walk around while you are picking up around the house, vacuuming, calling a friend to catch up, or watching your favorite show for 5–10 minutes. Moving this way can significantly improve your digestion and decrease bloating, or possibly eliminate it altogether.

31 Battle Bloating with Bitters

Herbal bitters are commonly used to help with digestion when it's not working as well as you'd like it to, usually as a result of a medical condition or a medication side effect. Bitters help by stimulating the secretion of your digestive enzymes and juices, which then aids in breaking down your food further and helps you avoid bloating. You can find many bitters products on the market that you can incorporate into your meals to help with digestion. When picking out which product will be best for you, consider where it's coming from, if it has been third-party tested, if there are positive reviews, the price point, and if you can tolerate the form it's in. Some bitters will come in liquid form and have a more distinct taste while others will be in capsule form.

Once you have your product of choice in hand, decide when to take it. Bitters usually will be most effective when taken just before your meal or within the first few bites of your meal. This allows them to get right to work increasing your enzyme and digestive juice levels as your food makes it to your stomach. Keep in mind that bitters will only work when taken with your meal, so for this intervention to give you relief from bloating, you have to take it regularly!

32 Find the Root Cause of Headaches

GLP-1 medications don't have a direct impact to trigger a headache, so if you are experiencing frequent headaches chances are it's something you are doing (or not doing) that's creating that pounding in your noggin. The main triggers of headaches while taking a GLP-1 are:

- Dehydration
- Electrolyte imbalances
- Protein deficiency
- Alcohol intake

Start by running through this list and ensuring that you're hydrated, you've got electrolytes on board, and you are eating enough protein each day. Odds are you can improve in at least one of these areas, so get to it! If you feel like you have all of these areas nailed down, it's possible that your headaches could correlate to your injections. Try tracking your headaches in a journal or note on your phone to see if you can determine a pattern around your injection day. Alcohol contributes to dehydration and also dilates blood vessels in your brain, which can trigger headaches. As a general rule, if you're struggling with headaches, avoiding alcohol and embracing mocktails can save you a world of pain and trouble.

If all else fails, seek out medical help from your healthcare professional to inquire about prescription medications and additional testing to get answers as to why your head won't leave you in peace.

33 Freeze Away Headaches

There's nothing quite like the feeling of an ice-cold cap sliding over your scalp while you have a raging headache. Cold intervention has been shown to significantly reduce headache (and even migraine) symptoms without any additional medications. There are actual caps for your head, typically made of gel or small ice packs sewn into a cap, that you can reuse over and over again. These mold to your head to provide direct cold therapy right to your brain.

Cold therapy can be done with the ice caps or with regular ice packs as long as you're able to surround your head with the cold. When coldness is applied to your head, it helps reduce inflammation and constrict your blood vessels, which can alleviate any pounding and prominent pain. The sensation of having freezing cold wrapped around your head can also provide a welcome distraction and even topical numbing from the cold to make the pain more bearable.

While there are relatively few risks with using a cold cap or cold therapy, there is naturally a risk of frostbite if you leave it on for too long, so be sure to follow the instructions of the ice cap you are using. Cold therapy can be an effective, inexpensive, and medication-free way to manage headache pain.

Bonus tip: If you don't want to buy a cold cap, you can DIY your own with ice packs and an ace bandage or a tight hat like a beanie and get a similar effect!

34 Avoid Hypoglycemia

Even if you didn't originally struggle with blood sugar levels, you can still experience hypoglycemia while taking a GLP-1 medication. Hypoglycemia refers to when you are having an episode of low blood sugar. This usually will feel like:

- Shaking
- Cold sweats
- Nausea
- Dizziness
- Increased heart rate
- Blurry vision
- Confusion

Hypoglycemia episodes can happen if you are going too long between meals, if you're not eating enough carbohydrates, or if you're not eating enough at your meals. Normally, when you eat a meal, your blood sugar naturally rises as you break down food and your GLP-1 medication helps your body regulate your blood sugar levels and insulin levels. However, while on your medicine, if you're not eating regularly it can create dips that are too low and your body will need you to intervene to get your blood sugar levels stable again.

To avoid hypoglycemia, you can follow a few rules:

- Eat a meal within 1 hour of waking up each day that's packed with 20–30 grams of protein.
- Have a small meal or snack every 3–4 hours after your first meal of the day.
- Create meals with a protein, a carbohydrate, and a fat component for balance.

By creating stability in your mealtimes along with balanced meals with protein and carbohydrates, you will have the best chance at avoiding hypoglycemia. If you find that you are having regular hypoglycemic episodes even with your best attempts at following these steps, consult with your healthcare provider for support.

35 Fix Hypoglycemia Fast

If you find yourself in a hypoglycemia episode, use the 15-15 rule and you will be able to raise your blood sugars right back up to normal. This rule can be used any time you are experiencing a confirmed low blood sugar episode or suspect you are having one. Here's how it works:

1 Eat or drink 15 grams of quick-acting carbohydrates.

2 Wait 15 minutes to reevaluate your symptoms and see how you're feeling.

3 Repeat every 15 minutes until your blood sugar levels have improved or your symptoms have resolved.

As a best practice, try to always keep some quick-acting carbohydrates on hand or near you. Quick-acting carbohydrates enter your bloodstream quickly to raise those glucose levels. Items that you can keep around in case you need to implement the 15-15 rule are:

- **Juices or sodas:** 4 ounces of regular soda (skip the diet soda; it won't help here) or juice equals one serving size (which equals about 15 grams).
- **Sugar and honey:** 1 tablespoon (which equals about 15 grams) of sugar, honey, or pure maple syrup can be used to raise blood sugar.
- **Candy:** Gummy candies, hard candies, and jelly beans can be used for quick help. The type of candy will determine how much to have; for example, Sour Patch Kids would be six to seven pieces to equal 15 grams of carbohydrates.
- **Glucose tablets:** These store-bought tablets are premeasured for easy access. Each brand will vary with how many tablets would equal 15 grams; be sure to read the instructions.
- **Glucose gels:** This is a store-bought gel, similar to tablets, that can travel easily. Follow the instructions on the individual product you buy.

36 | Feeling Helpless with Hair Loss

For many people, hair is a form of expression, something that they take pride in and spend a good amount of time and money maintaining, so when it starts falling out it can be a shock. Two primary triggers of hair loss include rapid weight loss and vitamin or mineral deficiencies. Unfortunately for GLP-1 users, both of these things can happen if you are not carefully monitoring your diet and weight loss.

Some people on GLP-1 medications see a slower weekly rate of weight loss but overall still lose a significant amount of body weight, whereas others can be hyper-responders who drop weight at a rapid pace that creates a substantial rate of weight loss in just a few months. This major change to body weight typically will start to show via hair loss around months three to four of taking your medication. By slowing down your weight loss or progressing at a slower pace on a lower dose, you can avoid some weight loss–related hair loss.

When you are taking GLP-1 medications, you can see a significant shift in the overall amount of food you are consuming and even the types of food you are able to tolerate when dealing with side effects. If your food intake drops too low, your fruit and vegetable intake decreases, or you stop eating your normal repertoire of foods, you can create unintentional deficiencies that can result in your hair shedding in excess. Ideally you should address any deficiencies in your food intake for the best results in the long term. Short term, you can add in a multivitamin or prenatal vitamin to help boost your nutrients, but remember, supplements should just be supplemental to your already adequate diet.

37 Slow Your Weight Loss

Weight loss is an end goal that so many share, but if it's not done safely and sustainably you'll end up paying the price later on. When thinking about a safe and sustainable rate of weight loss, consider the pace at which you can lose the weight without causing additional health issues (excess muscle loss, vitamin deficiencies, malnutrition) and the pace at which you will be able to maintain that weight loss over the long term.

With GLP-1 medications, weight can come off quickly, which is to be expected; however, there can be such a thing as *too quickly*. Without a GLP-1 medication, a sustainable rate of weight loss for the average person is about 1–2 pounds per week. Add in a GLP-1 medication, and you will see the same healthy pace or closer to the 2 pounds per week. It's worth noting that if you have over 100 pounds to lose, you may lose weight a bit quicker initially. Other factors like inflammation status and how often you exercise can also impact weight loss.

If you're seeing the weight come off for several consecutive months at a rapid pace and you're starting to notice you're having more side effects, are experiencing more fatigue, or are feeling weaker, it's time to slow down your weight loss. Here are a few helpful ideas for you:

- Do a quick calorie audit to see the amount at which you're currently eating, then focus on bumping up your calorie count from there.
- Consider a dose decrease with your medical provider.
- Add in resistance training to help preserve the muscle mass that you currently have.

38 Check Your Blood Work

Nutrient deficiencies and imbalances can occur while taking a GLP-1 medication. This is primarily due to the changes in your dietary intake as you navigate through no appetite, food aversions, changes to meal sizes, and lacking necessary nutrients and protein. If you are losing your hair or noticing changes in your nails and skin health, it's time to get your labs checked. In an ideal world, you can work with your healthcare provider and insurance company to get a full lab workup done to get a full picture to create the most comprehensive plan tailored to your individual needs. However, we don't always live in that ideal world.

Annually you should have a basic set of labs drawn. If you haven't had those recently you can request a:

- Comprehensive metabolic panel (CMP)
- Complete blood count (CBC)
- Hemoglobin A1C
- Lipid panel/profile (cholesterol, triglycerides, HDL, LDL)
- Vitamin D

Additional labs to request to get to the bottom of hair loss or changes to your nails and skin health are:

- Full thyroid panel (thyroid-stimulating hormone [TSH], free triiodothyronine [T3], total T3, reverse T3, free thyroxine [T4], total T4, thyroid peroxidase [TPO] and thyroglobulin [TgAb] antibodies)
- Vitamin B_{12}
- Vitamin A
- Zinc
- Magnesium
- Iron panel (iron, total iron-binding capacity [TIBC], ferritin, transferrin)

- Fasting insulin
- C-reactive protein
- Sex hormones (For women: estradiol, total estrogen, total testosterone, free testosterone, progesterone, dehydroepiandrosterone sulfate [DHEA-S], luteinizing hormone [LH], follicle-stimulating hormone [FSH], sex hormone-binding globulin [SHBG], pregnenolone, prolactin) (For men: testosterone [total and free], luteinizing hormone [LH], follicle-stimulating hormone [FSH], prolactin, and sex hormone-binding globulin [SHBG])

With a comprehensive list, you can work with your healthcare provider to get as many of these labs checked as possible to rule out any underlying issues that need additional attention.

39 Support Your Scalp

When your hair is falling out, it can also be a sign that your scalp is in distress. With a little extra tender loving care, you can support your scalp health while trying to get your hair loss to slow or stop completely. External care of your scalp and overall hair health can play a big role in helping to promote new hair growth to offset any hair loss.

Starting at the scalp, a primary intervention for your scalp health is going to be keeping a clean environment. If you have excess buildup of products like dry shampoo or oils, or even if you're just not rinsing your hair well enough, it can negatively impact the health of your scalp and your hair follicles. Aim to use a great clarifying shampoo, wash your hair regularly, and use dry shampoo or additional haircare products on your scalp sparingly. The second intervention you can consider adding in is a topical solution that supports scalp health and new hair growth. There are several scalp and hair oils on the market; you can take your pick of what fits your preference and budget.

You can also consider laser therapy, microneedling, or platelet-rich plasma injections that could help with new hair growth. Before jumping to these types of treatments though, you can also do little things to help with your hair habits. Try to avoid using excessive amounts of heat on your scalp and hair, avoid tight hairstyles that pull on your scalp, and use hairspray sparingly to avoid breakage.

40 Fight Fatigue

When you sign up to take a GLP-1 medication, fatigue is mentioned as a well-known side effect, but what you usually aren't told is that there's not really a concrete solution for it. Most of the time you just have to bide your time and ride out the fatigue as your body gets used to the GLP-1 medication. While that may be the case, you also can ensure that your habits are in the optimal spot to not worsen the fatigue. That's where this fighting fatigue checklist comes in. You can use this list to check off your habits to help limit your fatigue as much as possible while your body is adjusting.

To fight off fatigue try to:

- ☐ *Incorporate at least 10 minutes of walking or movement each day (bonus points if you are in natural sunlight!).*
- ☐ *Ensure you are getting at least 7 hours of quality sleep per night.*
- ☐ *Stay hydrated (dehydration is one of the most common reasons for daytime fatigue).*
- ☐ *Enjoy fresh air at least once per day for at least 30 minutes (you can break this into smaller time blocks if you need to).*
- ☐ *Monitor your caffeine intake; try to cap it around 200 milligrams per day.*
- ☐ *Limit your caffeine intake to before noon.*

41 Take the Extra Rest

As fatigue is a prevalent side effect for many GLP-1 users, especially for the first two to six weeks of starting the medication or of doing a dose increase, there are going to be times where extra rest can make a world of difference in how big of an impact that fatigue has on you.

There's not a one-size-fits-all way to determine if you should rest or push on, so it's going to be up to you to determine if you are just feeling like you are not up for something versus being tired enough to need an extra rest session. Here's a trick that you can use if you are trying to gauge if you need extra rest:

If you were to lie down in a dark, calm environment for 10–15 minutes, would you fall asleep? If the answer is yes, it's time to rest! If the answer is no, chances are you can push through and go crush any tasks that need your attention like cooking or going for a walk. If you do fall into the category of being able to fall asleep, close those eyes and get some extra rest. You deserve it, and your body does too!

42 Conquer Appetite Suppression

For some, appetite suppression can be an exciting new feeling, especially if they have always been plagued by consistent food noise that has led to temptation and feeling like they didn't have control over food. It can be refreshing to not think about your next meal or snack constantly, but you must be careful that it doesn't create a lack of awareness around ensuring you're eating meals regularly throughout the day. To make the most of your time on a GLP-1 medication, you can create a few lifestyle changes to help offset the appetite suppression.

Explore all these tips, or pick and choose which options are best for your own preferences and schedule:

- **Eat regular meals.** By scheduling out regular meals for yourself, you ensure you don't skip meals and cut your calories short. Regular meals throughout the day support a healthy metabolism and appetite.
- **Pick low-volume, high-calorie foods.** Instead of opting for low-calorie, high-volume foods, flip the script and aim for higher calorie density to help with your reduced portion capacity at meals. Instead of having cauliflower rice, for example, opt for regular rice. Keep snacks on hand like dried fruits for great nutrients and higher calorie density.
- **Add in exercise.** Regular exercise supports a healthy metabolism and can help with stimulating your appetite a bit.
- **Pick your favorite foods.** When you don't have a big appetite, including your favorite foods in your daily meals can help make mealtimes a bit more enticing. If you have several favorites, try to keep a rotation of them so that your lower appetite doesn't end up making you dislike a fan favorite.

43 Understand Hunger and Fullness Cues

One of the leading causes of nausea and vomiting while taking a GLP-1 medication is the inability to understand hunger and fullness cues. We all have normal and regular hunger cues to prompt us when it's time to eat, followed by fullness cues that tell us when we've eaten enough at meals. Hunger cues can become less reliable if you are undereating, experiencing high stress levels, adding in a new medication, or aren't sleeping well.

GLP-1 medications silence your hunger cues and therefore you won't be able to rely on your body automatically letting you know it's time for more food. This lack of hunger cues can also lead you to go for hours without a meal and then quickly consume too much food and end up uncomfortably full.

When you eat any meal, whether on a GLP-1 medication or not, your body gradually starts to fill up and slowly over time your brain gets signals that you are full. While taking a GLP-1 medication, chances are you are going to actually be full long before the signal reaches your brain since your stomach capacity is lower. So if you are not being told naturally to eat anymore and you can't always trust if you are full enough, what can you do to create stability for yourself?

You can create your own hunger and fullness system. You are going to proactively plan to have a meal or snack every few hours to avoid feeling sick. While you are eating your meals, you are going to slow down the pace and start with smaller portions on your plate to be able to evaluate if you really want to eat more, and then go back for seconds if you do! By creating your own system you should be able to avoid any nausea or vomiting.

44 Use Strategic Eating, Not Intuitive Eating

Intuitive eating has become a popular topic in recent years as more people want to reject restrictive ways of eating. It's also become quite popular to use "intuitive eating" to lose weight without having to pay attention to specific calories or foods. Unfortunately, there's nothing intuitive about weight loss, so true intuitive eating that follows your body's natural hunger and fullness cues isn't possible when aiming to lose weight.

GLP-1 medications and true intuitive eating also do not go hand in hand. Because your natural hunger cues are muted while taking GLP-1s, and your fullness cues are being altered due to slower digestion, you no longer have natural cues to follow.

The great news is that you don't have to jump from intuitive eating to the opposite end of the spectrum where you track every single piece of food you eat and every sip you drink. If you prefer intuitive eating over food tracking, you can instead implement *strategic eating*. To strategically eat, you can follow this framework:

- Aim to have a meal every 3–4 hours throughout the day.
- Add a fruit or vegetable, paired with a carbohydrate/starch source, and a protein to all your meals.
- When eating your meals, work through your plate in the order of protein first, then fruits and vegetables, finishing with your carbohydrate source.

This framework allows you to still have control over your meal and food choices, while prioritizing your important nutrient needs and avoiding undereating.

45 Improve Sagging Skin

Some people on GLP-1 medications can lose over half their body weight. With major weight loss comes significant changes to your skin and its elasticity. Every body is different, but there are several main factors that can lead to excess or sagging skin after losing weight on GLP-1 medications.

- **Weight loss rate.** With rapid weight loss, body composition changes quickly. When the body shrinks considerably in a short period of time, your skin cannot match the pace to shrink with it.

- **Age.** As you age, you don't have the same elasticity and collagen production, which can make it a slower process for the skin to adapt and, in some cases, skin may not fully return to match the current size of the body.

- **Genetics.** Genetics heavily influences where you store fat on your body. Your individual fat stores and where most of your weight has come off your body can also heavily influence excess skin presence.

Depending on your own body and how much extra skin you have, there are several options for seeing improvement in the physical appearance of excess skin.

- If you lost weight quickly but it was a moderate amount of weight, over time, with patience, your skin likely will catch up most if not all of the way and return to a normal appearance.

- Hydration is a major component to having healthy, radiant, and elastic skin, so staying hydrated can support your skin recovering.

- Resistance training is also a great way to continue modifying your body composition, and filling out your body with more muscle can help with the appearance of skin.

Of course, time will be the most helpful natural intervention to see changes to your skin.

46 Surviving Sulfur Burps

One of the less common side effects while taking GLP-1 medications are the dreaded sulfur burps. Because sulfur burps are burps that taste and smell like rotten eggs, if you have them you may feel a bit panicked that something is wrong. Sometimes hydrogen sulfide gas can be produced in your gastrointestinal tract; if that happens and you burp (burping can be normal), it comes with a pungent smell.

When food is sitting in your gastrointestinal tract for longer periods of time, as it can when you are taking a GLP-1 medication, this can lead to an increased risk of sulfur burps. As the food sits, hydrogen sulfide gas can be produced. Most people report that sulfur burps are only around for a short period of time, usually when they are starting a new GLP-1 or after a dose increase. To help decrease their impact on your life, you can make two adjustments:

- Break your meals into smaller portions (if they're already small, go even smaller) so that you can digest your food and have less food sitting in your digestive system at once.
- Reduce intake of foods that are rich in sulfur for the short term until symptoms resolve (for example, cruciferous vegetables, garlic, onions, eggs, red meat, and so on).

If sulfur burps continue, you can consult your healthcare provider for medication support to manage them until they pass.

3 | Nutrition Blueprint

With a diet rich in lean protein, fruits, vegetables, whole grains, and healthy fats, there's almost nothing that can stop you. However, the Standard American Diet tends to lack fruits, vegetables, and protein, and run high in saturated fats, sugar, and carbohydrates. When you are on your GLP-1 medication, you will need to be aware that you may have to make big changes to your diet. GLP-1 medications will require you to be more precise with your macronutrient and micronutrient intake so you can achieve the maximum health benefits you're looking for.

When you're making major changes to your dietary intake, it can be confusing and overwhelming to know how to do it or what advice to follow. This chapter will take you through a blueprint of what vitamins and minerals are important to stay on top of while taking your medication, how to increase protein intake with actionable recommendations, and how to improve the overall quality of your diet to be able to live your happiest and healthiest life.

47 | Optimize Your Vitamin Intake

While it is always important to stay on top of your vitamin intake, it is even more important when taking a GLP-1 medication. Because these medications can impact your appetite and support you being in a calorie deficit, they can put you at an increased risk of nutrient deficiencies.

Vitamins are considered micronutrients. Without micronutrients your body would struggle to perform daily functions. Micronutrients are critical for the proper working of your immune system, signaling pathways throughout your body, enzyme production and function, antioxidant support, and more. Without micronutrients you can experience symptoms such as increased fatigue, hair loss, brittle nails, dry skin, and decreased mental clarity, to name a few. When a GLP-1 medication is added into your routine, it can lead to decreased food intake, which can quickly lead to decreased micronutrient intake and increased risk of deficiencies.

It's ideal to get your vitamin intake from food sources, so you may need to be more aware and methodical in your meal planning to be sure you're not shortchanging yourself. To make this as easy as possible, follow the 4:2 minimum rule: four vegetables and two fruits per day at a *minimum*. While micronutrients don't only come from fruits or vegetables, these two food groups are the ones that are most commonly missed, so being proactive and counting your portions of each can help create a strong foundation for your vitamin intake. If possible, you can always aim to eat *more* than four servings of vegetables and two servings of fruit, to optimize your vitamin intake further.

48 | Avoid Vitamin D Deficiency

You may have heard that getting into the sun more can help support your vitamin D intake, which is true, but it's important to know how else you can get this important vitamin without sitting in the sun. Vitamin D plays a role in your cognitive health, heart health, bone health, and immune function, and it can be a piece of the hair loss puzzle (see Feeling Helpless with Hair Loss in the previous chapter). In addition, when people taking a GLP-1 undereat and cause a vitamin D deficiency, they can suffer fatigue, feel muscle weakness, and negatively impact their brain/cognitive functions.

You can monitor your body for possible signs that you're not getting enough vitamin D. Fatigue, bone or joint pain, muscle weakness, hair loss, or even changes to mood can be associated with a deficiency. There are multiple food sources that have been fortified with vitamin D (fortified means during the manufacturing process the food has vitamin D added to it) like breakfast cereals, milk alternatives, or milk. Vitamin D can also be found in fatty fish (tuna, mackerel, salmon, trout), egg yolks, beef liver, and cheese.

To increase your vitamin D levels, aim to incorporate a variety of food sources, whether natural or fortified, in your daily food intake. If certain food sources are off the table because of preference or dietary restrictions, you could consider supplementation and work with your healthcare provider to determine what's best for you. Individual supplement needs will vary depending on your dietary intake and should be paired with your current vitamin D levels that your provider can check to determine your optimal path to healthy vitamin D levels.

49 Care About Calcium

Calcium helps with blood clotting, muscles contracting, your heart beating, healthy bones, and your nerves firing. If your calcium intake falls short, your body will actually take calcium from your bones to use in your bloodstream, which over long periods of time can lead to major negative ramifications for bone health.

GLP-1 medications can create major changes to your food intake and changes in the foods you eat. This can create a decrease in calcium intake that can negatively impact your bone health. In addition, along with the weight loss that occurs when taking GLP-1 medications can come muscle loss, which creates a higher risk for weakened bones.

Calcium and vitamin D work together; if you are deficient in vitamin D, you could become deficient in calcium. Calcium needs vitamin D to be absorbed into your body, so the pair needs to be kept together in good standing for optimal health. Low calcium can present as scaly dry skin, brittle nails, changes to your hair, increased muscle cramps, or muscle aches.

To prevent a calcium deficiency and your body taking calcium from your bones, you can focus on incorporating foods that are rich in calcium such as:

- Dairy products like yogurt, kefir, milk, and cheese
- Tofu
- Sardines and salmon
- Fortified juices like orange or grapefruit
- Fortified almond or rice milk
- Cooked vegetables like collard greens, spinach, kale, lamb's quarters, nettles, amaranth leaves

Daily requirements for intake of calcium change throughout life. Generally, for adults 19–50 years old, 1,000 milligrams per day is recommended. Always consult your healthcare provider for your specific intake recommendations.

50 Stay Energized with Vitamin B$_{12}$

B$_{12}$ is a crucial vitamin that you want to be sure you are getting enough of, especially when taking a GLP-1 medication. Vitamin B$_{12}$ is essential for cell metabolism, nerve function, hair health, red blood cell formation, and DNA production, and it might even help with side effects of GLP-1 medications like nausea and fatigue. Whether or not you are taking a GLP-1, if you don't have enough B$_{12}$ in your system, you're more likely to experience fatigue, weakness, hair loss, numbness and tingling in your extremities, and memory or cognition issues.

Vitamin B$_{12}$ needs can typically be met via daily food intake, so when taking a GLP-1 medication you'll want to be sure that you keep a regular rotation of B$_{12}$-rich foods in your food arsenal. Common side effects of GLP-1 medications like hair loss, fatigue, and nausea can all be worsened without proper B$_{12}$ levels. To prevent these side effects from low B$_{12}$ intake, you can focus on eating animal products such as clams, mussels, mackerel, salmon, crab, lean beef, beef liver, low-fat milk or yogurt, cheese, or eggs. Fortified milks or cereals can also be great options for B$_{12}$ intake.

If you are vegetarian or vegan, you are more likely to have a B$_{12}$ deficiency as many sources of this vitamin are found in animal products. B$_{12}$ levels can also be depleted more quickly in those with additional health conditions like polycystic ovary syndrome (PCOS) or autoimmune conditions, so for some, supplementation may be needed.

51 | Find Your Folate (Vitamin B₉)

If weakness, fatigue, shortness of breath, hair loss, or brain fog resonate with how you're feeling, you may be short on vitamin B_9, aka folate. Folate is slightly different from folic acid (another form of B_9) in that *folate* is naturally found in foods while *folic acid* is manufactured and then used as a supplement or added to foods to fortify them. When taking your GLP-1 medication, to prevent hair loss or fatigue, or to prevent those side effects from worsening, you'll want to focus on keeping folate-rich foods in your refrigerator.

Some of the best food sources of folate are dark leafy greens and fruits. Brussels sprouts, broccoli, spinach, lettuce, or asparagus can be great options for folate. In addition to fruits and vegetables, sunflower seeds, peanuts, whole grains, and beans can also be great additions to stock up on for folate intake. If your food preferences don't lean heavily toward dark leafy greens, try to hide them in smoothies or sauces to "sneak" them in. If even hiding them in your normal dishes doesn't work, you may need to pivot to fortified foods to get your daily recommended intake. Look for pastas, breads, rice, or breakfast cereals that have been fortified with folic acid to help increase your folate intake. Before resorting to supplements for folate, give it your best effort to get your intake via food for the best health outcomes.

52 Eat Your Vitamin K

When you think of vitamin K, you may think of its role in blood clotting, as that's what it's known most for, or perhaps you've heard of the health benefits of taking a combination vitamin D and K supplement. It's important to get enough vitamin K daily to support your GLP-1 journey as vitamin K can help support a healthy insulin response and healthy blood sugar levels when you have adequate intake.

Vitamin K is also one of the easier vitamins to get through your food intake. Two fruits that are great for vitamin K intake are grapes and kiwis. Kiwi is also wonderful for constipation relief (which can be a common side effect with GLP-1s), so it delivers a double whammy. Leafy greens like spinach, kale, collards, and broccoli are all good sources of vitamin K. You can also find vitamin K in many common foods like edamame, carrots, figs, pine nuts, and blueberries.

Here are three recipe ideas for you to get your daily vitamin K:

- Combine steamed edamame with some sea salt and chili oil and serve as a spicy side dish, if you can handle spice.
- Make a salad of kale and spinach (or your favorite greens); add blueberries, pine nuts, goat cheese, and a vinaigrette dressing.
- Drizzle some chopped kale with olive oil and sea salt and then roast in the oven for a crunchy snack.

53 | Choose Vitamin C–Rich Foods for Protection

Vitamin C is a powerful antioxidant that helps protect you and your cells from damage that can be caused by oxidative stress. It helps support energy levels, hair health, and immune function. One of the leading causes of a vitamin C deficiency is a poor-quality diet. Most people rely on their dietary intake to get adequate vitamin C to prevent deficiencies, but if your diet is lacking in fruits and vegetables, you're not setting yourself up for success. When you are deficient in vitamin C you can have poorer health outcomes and can experience hair loss or fatigue at higher levels while on a GLP-1, so be mindful of your intake to avoid those side effects. To support yourself on your GLP-1 medication, aim to keep a regular rotation of vitamin C–rich foods in your meals.

While oranges are a good source of vitamin C, they aren't actually the best source. There are several other fruits and vegetables that pack a bigger vitamin C punch. Kakadu plums, acerola cherries, rose hips, chili peppers, guava, yellow bell peppers, cantaloupe, parsley, mustard spinach, kale, kiwis, broccoli, Brussels sprouts, lychee, papaya, and strawberries are all excellent sources of vitamin C. If you rotate through a variety of these sources, you'll get an excellent intake of vitamin C plus great fiber as well.

54 Explore Vitamin E

Vitamin E is an antioxidant that fights free radicals in the body to prevent damage to your cells. The excellent news about vitamin E is that you're likely getting enough in your dietary intake. However, when taking a GLP-1 medication, it is possible that when changing your food intake, your vitamin E consumption can decline. Since vitamin E protects cells from damage and supports reproductive health, immune function, vision, and skin health, it's important to not drop the ball on your dietary intake.

With a bit of intention in your day, you can ensure that your diet supplies enough vitamin E. Seeds, nuts, fruits, vegetables, and even plant-based oils can provide your necessary vitamin E intake. Occasionally you may see oils getting a bad reputation, but sunflower, safflower, and soybean oil all provide vitamin E, which is supportive of your health. Avocados, sunflower seeds, peanuts, peanut butter, asparagus, collard greens, spinach, pumpkin, red bell peppers, butternut squash, and mangoes also are great sources of vitamin E.

To mix up a quick vitamin E–packed snack, create a small chopped salad with an avocado, a raw red bell pepper, and some spinach and drizzle with a bit of olive oil, salt, and pepper. If you're in the mood for something sweeter, you can try roasted butternut squash with a peanut butter drizzle and a sprinkle of cinnamon to create a side dish or snack that's rich in vitamin E!

55 | Remember Your Iron

Temporary aversions to protein or meats can be a common experience for those taking a GLP-1, as can food intake dropping too low. This creates the perfect storm for you to become iron deficient. When you don't take in enough iron, you are more likely to experience fatigue, which could keep you from feeling your best on your GLP-1 journey. Unfortunately, taking iron supplements can make other side effects (like constipation) worse, so it's best to get your iron intake from food.

Iron supplementation can work against you in two ways:

- Constipation typically accompanies iron supplementation, and if you're already battling constipation from your GLP-1 medication, you can get severely constipated very quickly.
- You could over supplement with iron and create toxic levels in your body that can be dangerous to your overall health.

If you need to supplement, be sure to have your healthcare provider oversee your dosages.

Rather than supplement with iron, you should pack your diet with iron-rich foods. Shellfish (clams, oysters, mussels, shrimp), liver and organ meats, red meat, turkey, legumes, tofu, spinach, quinoa, dark chocolate, and pumpkin seeds can all provide adequate amounts of iron when consumed regularly.

For a tasty treat, you can take pumpkin seeds and drizzle them with dark chocolate and a bit of sea salt for a good dose of iron. Enjoy straight out of the refrigerator or freezer for the best experience.

56 Experience the Healing Power of Zinc

Zinc is a necessary mineral to have as your body doesn't make zinc on its own. Zinc supplements are commonly pushed for immune support especially if you are sick, but if you take too much zinc long term, which is a good possibility with supplementing regularly, you can actually block the absorption of other minerals, like copper. Not having enough copper in your system can create a whole different set of health issues. So rather than supplement, you should focus on food intake for your zinc support.

Zinc is important for your overall immune function and, like GLP-1 medications, it also helps reduce inflammation in your body. For zinc-rich foods, you have two main categories to choose from: meat and seafood sources or plant-based sources. Seafood like oysters, crab, and lobster are rich in zinc. Beef and pork are also great options for zinc intake. Plant sources include chickpeas, legumes (kidney beans), nuts (cashews), oats, tofu, and seeds (hempseeds, pumpkin seeds).

For most people, consuming too much zinc via food is highly unlikely; eating foods rich in zinc is a safe way to get enough of this important mineral. If you find yourself needing to supplement zinc, be sure to work with your healthcare provider to oversee your blood levels to avoid excess supplementation.

57 | Maximize Your Magnesium

Magnesium is a participant in over three hundred reactions in the body. Without adequate magnesium, you can experience muscle cramps, muscle weakness, fatigue, low appetite, and nausea. These side effects of low magnesium can be difficult to manage under usual circumstances, but when you add a GLP-1 medication, it typically leads to increased instances of feeling exhausted and nauseated. Thankfully, you can boost your magnesium intake naturally with specific foods.

To quickly increase your magnesium levels, you'll want to aim to incorporate magnesium-rich foods in almost all, if not all, of your meals each day. Leafy greens, seeds, nuts, legumes, and whole grains are great magnesium sources. An example day of eating with magnesium-rich foods could look like:

- **Breakfast:** chia seed pudding
- **Lunch:** spinach salad with your protein of choice
- **Dinner:** taco salad with black beans, rice, and kidney beans
- **Snacks:** banana with peanut butter, apple with yogurt

Magnesium supplements are also generally considered safe for most people to use, so if you do find that you're not able to increase your levels naturally through diet alone, you may want to consider a magnesium chloride or magnesium glycinate supplement (always check with your healthcare provider first). There's always the chance of magnesium toxicity with supplementation, so proceed with caution and only use it when necessary and with medical supervision.

58 Get Your Omega-3s from Fish

Omega-3 fatty acids are polyunsaturated fats that you need as an essential part of your daily dietary intake. Your body cannot make enough omega-3 fatty acids on its own, so you can bridge the gap by ensuring your diet is rich in omega-3s. With adequate omega-3 intake, you may lower your risk for cardiovascular disease and blood clots. Without adequate omega-3 intake, you're likely to experience dry skin, increased acne, dry eyes, mood changes, joint pain, or hair loss. Taking a GLP-1 medication increases the importance of getting adequate omega-3s to maintain healthy cholesterol levels and avoid hair loss as a side effect of the GLP-1.

There are three main types of omega-3 fatty acids (eicosapentaenoic acid [EPA], docosahexaenoic acid [DHA], and alpha-linolenic acid [ALA]), and two of them (EPA and DHA) are easy to obtain through marine sources. Fatty fish like salmon, mackerel, tuna, sardines, and herring all have high omega-3 content per serving. Shellfish, tilapia, cod, and bass also are marine sources of omega-3s; however, they're not as fatty so the EPA and DHA content is lower.

The quickest way to eat enough fish to satisfy your EPA and DHA needs would be to choose one of the fattier fishes and have two to three servings per week to meet your overall dietary needs without supplementation. It can be as easy as eating salmon two or three times a week with a portion size of 3–4 ounces each time.

If there's no chance you will become a regular fish consumer, you'll want to focus on getting your omega-3 fatty acids using ALA sources, which are plant based, and also consult with your healthcare provider about an omega-3 supplement that will be best for you.

59 | Source Your Omega-3s from Plants

Alpha-linolenic acid (ALA) is the omega-3 fatty acid that is found in plant sources. It's not produced naturally in your body, so you have to rely on your intake via food sources. Ideally, you should incorporate a variety of plant sources rich in ALA to create a diverse diet and also consume adequate amounts of ALA.

Food sources of ALA can include flaxseed, chia seeds, walnuts, hempseeds, soybeans, spinach, and Brussels sprouts. Here are some ideas for incorporating these foods into your day:

- Walnuts can easily be incorporated in your oatmeal, baked goods, as a solo snack, on a snack platter, or tossed in your granola mix for a great omega-3–packed crunch.
- Flaxseed, chia seeds, or hempseeds can easily be incorporated as sprinkles on top of your dishes or blended into your smoothies or even soups.
- If you're looking for an idea to incorporate more soybeans for ALA, try adding them to your chili or soup recipes.

If you're unable to tolerate or consume the other marine sources of omega-3s (EPA and DHA), you'll likely want to consider supplementing your diet with an omega-3 supplement to ensure you are getting enough daily. You'll want to choose a high-quality supplement with the support of your healthcare provider that best meets your needs.

60 Aim for Healthy Sources of Omega-6s

Omega-6 fatty acids tend to have a bad reputation. However, in recent years, there have been updates and new information that shine a light on the more positive side of omega-6 fatty acid intake.

That's not to say that you want to go wild and overdo your omega-6 intake, but rather you can live more in the middle and know that omega-6s can be helpful, but in some cases can still potentially cause inflammation. On the positive side, omega-6 fatty acids can help lower LDL cholesterol (harmful cholesterol), boost HDL (helpful cholesterol), improve insulin sensitivity, reduce heart disease, and reduce inflammation.

The average diet for adults includes plenty of omega-6 fatty acids, so it's rare that you would be deficient on a daily basis; however, to optimize your health, especially when on your GLP-1 medication, try to aim for healthier sources of omega-6s. You can try boosting your intake of walnuts, sunflower seeds, tofu, eggs, and almonds for great omega-6s paired with some additional micronutrients and protein. You can also find great omega-6s in safflower oil and canola oil. Use caution in foods that are higher in saturated fats, even if they have a good amount of omega-6 fatty acids in them; saturated fat adds up quickly and can contribute to poorer health outcomes when consumed in excess.

61 Balance Your Omega-6–Rich Foods

With the discourse changing around omega-6 fatty acid intake, it's still important that you get a healthy balance of omega-6–rich foods paired with omega-3–rich foods so that you don't overconsume in the omega-6 category. When taking a GLP-1 medication, one of the foundational pieces of success is to have balanced nutrient intake to prevent side effects, improve health markers, and support your weight loss journey. Most adults consume far more omega-6 fatty acids in their diet and shortchange their omega-3 intake. If you're unsure on where you land between the two, you can start by evaluating how many omega-3s you take in on a daily basis. If you are short on omega-3s, start by increasing your omega-3 intake before trying to restrict your omega-6s to improve that balance. If you are already getting sufficient omega-3s regularly, you can reduce your omega-6 intake to improve the balance between the two.

What if you're not sure how many omega-6 fatty acids you're consuming overall? You can simply track your food intake for just a few days to get a better idea. A quick and relatively easy way to do this would be with Cronometer, a free tracking app you can download to your phone. It allows you to track your fat intake and also shows you the ratio between your omega-3s and omega-6s. While food tracking isn't for everyone, if you truly aren't sure where your omega-6 intake is at or where you're landing ratio-wise, it is a very helpful tool; in about seven days you can collect an average data picture. This allows you to tailor your dietary intake to what you specifically need to optimize your omega-6 intake.

62 Understand How Calories Impact Metabolism

A common misconception that can derail your progress on your GLP-1 medication is the idea that the calories you take in don't impact your metabolism and you can simply rely on your GLP-1 medication to overrule your metabolism. You cannot outwork your metabolism with a GLP-1 medication. You may be able to see a bit more weight loss while on a GLP-1 than if you weren't taking one, but eventually your metabolism will catch up to you if you don't sustainably tackle your weight loss on your GLP-1.

When you are restricting your calories while on a GLP-1 medication, over time your metabolism will adapt to your current calorie intake. This will require you to adjust your calorie targets to continue seeing progress, but eventually you will hit a plateau that not even calorie reduction can break. This is your metabolism and your body's way of telling you that if you want to lose more weight, you're going to need a break from dieting.

So how can you avoid this? To keep your calories in a safe range, you'll want to start by figuring out your total daily energy expenditure, or TDEE (see the following entry). From there, you will be able to safely start a calorie deficit of 15–20 percent and then as you plateau (defined as three to four weeks minimum with no progress but 90 percent adherence to habits), you can work up to a 30 percent calorie deficit. When you eventually plateau at the 30 perfect deficit point, you likely won't be able to safely take more calories away without creating unnecessary risk to your health, and you will need a break from dieting. When this happens, you will want to reverse your diet back up to a maintenance level of calories and spend multiple months there.

63 Calculate Your Calorie Needs

If you want to experience the best results for weight loss on your GLP-1, or you just want to understand your body's calorie needs better, it's time to grab your calculator. For the average adult, the Mifflin-St. Jeor equation is one of the most widely used predictive equations for estimating calorie needs; it measures your resting metabolic rate. There's an equation for females and males to calculate based on biological sex. To figure out your daily calorie needs, you enter your individual measurements (weight, height, and age) into the equation and then factor in your activity level with the corresponding multiplier.

Start with the applicable Mifflin-St. Jeor equation:

FEMALES

$$(10 \times \text{weight [in kg]}) + (6.25 \times \text{height [in cm]}) - (5 \times \text{age [years]}) - 161$$

MALES

$$(10 \times \text{weight [in kg]}) + (6.25 \times \text{height [in cm]}) - (5 \times \text{age [years]}) + 5$$

Next, you'll determine your activity level and factor in that multiplier by applying it to your result from the Mifflin-St. Jeor equation. There are five activity levels. You'll want to *honestly* gauge your activity level for the best accuracy:

- **Sedentary:** Multiply by 1.2 (this would be minimal activity)
- **Light activity:** Multiply by 1.375 (about one to two workouts per week, and around 5,000 steps on average per day)
- **Moderate activity:** Multiply by 1.55 (about three to five workouts per week, and around 5,000–10,000 steps on average per day)

- **Active:** Multiply by 1.725 (about five workouts or more per week, and around 10,000 or more steps on average per day)
- **Very Active:** Multiply by 1.9 (typically for elite athletes or specific situations)

You'll likely be somewhere between the light and moderate activity ranges while taking your GLP-1 medication. Once you multiply your Mifflin-St. Jeor number by your activity factor, you'll have your overall total daily energy expenditure (TDEE), also known as your maintenance calories.

64 | Find the Best Calorie-Counting Fit

Counting calories can be a great educational tool in your overall weight loss toolkit, and the process can be highly customized to you and your lifestyle. Some may need to be more general with calorie counting; others may want to be as precise as tracking down the number of grams of a specific macronutrient. It's important to pick a method that is going to be realistic and sustainable for your life and schedule.

When deciding how specific you'd like to get with your calorie counting, start by assessing your:

- Experience with tracking
- Resources to be able to track (digital scale, measuring cups, tracking apps)
- Time available in your schedule to measure out your food and track it
- Personal feelings and bias toward food tracking

How can you decide how specific you should get? If you are someone who has never tracked before and is brand-new to tracking, you likely will have the most success with overall calorie counting. If you have some tracking experience and want to be a bit more precise with your tracking, you could consider tracking overall calories and a protein goal. If you have previous experience tracking, you can typically have the most optimal outcomes by tracking down to the grams with macronutrients.

When it comes to finding the best fit for how specific you should get with keeping track of your calorie intake, you will always want to go with what feels best for you; there's no one size fits all. There can be negative feelings or habits that can come with calorie tracking, and if that's you, be sure to take a step back and evaluate if you can safely track your intake.

65 Evaluate Your Macronutrients and Micronutrients

Let's dive into the nitty-gritty of nutrition, not just calories, but macronutrients versus micronutrients. Overall, your dietary intake includes grams of protein, carbohydrates, and fats, known as macronutrients. Plus, vitamins and minerals like vitamin C, sodium, potassium, and so on, known as micronutrients.

You need a combination of both macronutrients and micronutrients to create a well-rounded diet to support your optimal health. When taking a GLP-1 medication, macronutrient and micronutrient intake becomes even more important to help prevent or manage side effects, prevent muscle loss, support fat loss, and reduce inflammation. Micronutrient needs will vary from person to person, but a great place to start would be to evaluate how your current micronutrient intake stacks up against the recommended daily intake. For macronutrients, ideally you should aim to have your protein intake be between 20–25 percent of your total calories, carbohydrates between 45–65 percent of your total calories, and fats 20–35 percent of your total calories.

Here's how you can quickly check your daily macronutrient balance:

1 Calculate your total grams of carbohydrates consumed and multiply by 4 to get your total calories from carbohydrates; divide that number by your total calorie goal; then multiply by 100.

2 Calculate your total grams of protein consumed and multiply by 4 to get your total calories from protein; divide that number by your total calorie goal; then multiply by 100.

3 Calculate your total grams of fats consumed and multiply by 9 to get your total calories from fats; divide that number by your total calorie goal; then multiply by 100.

Now that you have your percentage for carbohydrates, protein, and fats, you can compare them to the recommended ranges provided to ensure you're falling within range.

66 | Eat Your Protein

There are three magic words when it comes to nutrition and your GLP-1 journey: Eat your protein.

While it may seem silly to say that protein is a magical fix, it can solve many of the side effects or negative outcomes that can come with GLP-1 medications. Muscle loss, for example, happens during any weight loss journey, but it occurs in greater amounts without adequate daily protein intake. Low protein intake can also increase fatigue, worsen nausea, and lead to hair loss—all of which can happen while taking a GLP-1 medication. Fortunately, these problems can be prevented or minimized with adequate protein intake.

Chances are, if you've never tracked your protein intake, or aren't doing that currently, you're likely underestimating your protein intake. So how do you know what you need to eat at a minimum for protein? You can do a quick calculation yourself or book a visit with a dietitian for customized help. If you want to find a protein starting point by yourself, you can use the following calculation: Take your body weight in pounds and divide it by 2.2 to convert it to kilograms. Then multiply your weight in kilograms by 1 gram per kilogram for your minimum protein goal. In other words, your weight in kilograms is equal to the minimum number of grams of protein you should eat every day. One caveat: If you have a very high current body weight, this equation may give you an unrealistically high protein goal. Instead, calculate what 15 percent of your overall total daily energy expenditure (TDEE) is and divide it by 4 to get your protein minimum goal (example: if your TDEE is 2200, 15 percent would be 330 calories, divided by 4, which would be a minimum of 83 grams of protein per day).

If you are wanting to lose weight on your GLP-1, aim for a protein intake of at least 20–25 percent of your overall calorie intake.

67 | Increase Your Protein Intake

You know protein intake is important, but it might not be second nature to you, and it might feel like you're having to put every ounce of mental energy toward getting your protein in. It may even feel like you're spending more time thinking about protein than you are about anything else throughout the day. The good news is that you don't have to keep feeling like this.

By implementing a few safeguards into your daily routine, you can add opportunities for protein without too much hassle. Set yourself up for success by first ensuring regular mealtimes where you have 20–30 grams of protein at each meal, with a minimum of three meals per day. This allows you to get at least 60–90 grams of protein without any additional snacks or meals.

Second, aim to keep quick protein-packed snacks on deck when you're out and about. This could be a protein shake, protein bar, or jerky, or you might grab some hard-boiled eggs, a Greek yogurt cup, or a protein-focused snack at a drive-through (think grilled nuggets or egg bites).

Third, prioritize protein on your plate. With your meal size decreasing on GLP-1 medications and becoming fuller faster, you'll want to focus on the protein on your plate first. Once your protein is gone, move on to the rest of your dish. This ensures that you still get your protein in the event that you're too full to finish the full meal.

68 Quick Fixes for Extra Protein

Even with your best planning and preparation to get all your required protein each day, it's possible that you may come up short and need a boost. If you can keep some quick protein-packed options on hand for those moments, you'll have a better chance of not falling short. Protein is a satiating food, meaning it helps keep you fuller longer, and, as you know, your GLP-1 medication also helps keep you feeling fuller longer. So it's likely that you will be needing smaller chunks of protein throughout the day.

To add in extra protein without adding extra volume, you can try:

- Swapping out some of your eggs for egg whites, or adding egg whites to your mixture
- Adding cottage cheese to your egg mixture
- Swapping in Greek yogurt for regular yogurt

For a quick protein boost, you can try:

- Jerky
- Chicken, tuna, or salmon packets (on average, one pack is four to six bites and 13–19 grams of protein)
- Edamame
- Turkey or chicken roll ups
- Hard-boiled eggs
- Protein shakes (powdered or premade)

If you are at a point in your day where you don't have a ton of physical room left for more food without becoming uncomfortably full, you will want to aim for a lower-volume option to get more protein in. This could be an 8-ounce protein shake, or a chicken packet, or a small yogurt cup. If you have more room, try combining a few sources of protein or increase the serving size to get closer to your overall protein goal.

69 | Preplan Your Protein

One of the quickest and easiest ways to make sure you're getting enough protein intake through your day is to incorporate animal proteins. Animal protein can include the typical chicken, eggs, turkey, dairy products, beef, pork, fish, and seafood and also less common sources like bison, elk, deer, or even alligator. Even with an abundance of options in animal proteins, most people average too little protein daily. To avoid this low-protein problem, you can create a preferred protein list that includes your easy (and enjoyable) protein picks.

Start by making a list on paper or on your phone of all the protein sources you like. An example list could be: ground chicken, chicken breast, chicken thighs, ground turkey, salmon, tilapia, cod, pork, yogurt, shrimp, eggs, egg whites. Once you have your list of protein options you like, then go ahead and create a second list of two to three different ways you enjoy preparing or eating that protein (example: scrambled eggs, egg bites, egg tacos). These two lists will give you multiple options for several different protein choices. This will allow you to pick and choose among various proteins, varying the type, taste, and preparation.

The more variety you have in your protein sources, the easier it will be to consistently hit your protein intake goal and avoid burning out on one specific protein source. The last step here to really make things easy for yourself is to preplan your week and slot in one protein source per meal, with at least three meals per day.

70 Try Plants for Protein

When you think of adding protein to your diet, like most people you probably automatically jump right to animal sources, which are a great way to get your protein. However, you may not want to eat animal protein, have allergies to some animal proteins, or prefer to follow a more plant-based approach to eating. Even if you enjoy animal protein, having a variety of protein sources while taking your GLP-1 medication is important for overall microbiome support and fiber intake.

Plant-based protein sources include beans, legumes, edamame, chickpeas, lentils, nuts, seeds, quinoa, soy milk, seitan, tempeh, tofu, oats, nut butters, sorghum, peas, nutritional yeast, and other meat substitutes like meatless burger patties or sausages.

To successfully implement plant-based proteins in your diet, you'll want to aim to have a variety of different sources throughout the day. An important fact to remember is that seitan, tofu, tempeh, and edamame are typically higher in protein than grain sources like oats or rice, so creating a daily rotation of higher-protein plant options will be essential to getting enough protein overall. Aim to incorporate a higher-protein option in all three main meals of your day and add in the other plant-based protein sources as snacks and sides to complement your main protein.

71 Balance Your Carbohydrates

Carbohydrate intake can come from a variety of sources like fruits, vegetables, and grains. They're also often found in highly processed foods such as pastries, white breads, candy, chips, and sugary cereals. Without intention behind your carbohydrate choices, you may find that the majority of your carbohydrate intake is coming from the more processed sources; this isn't inherently bad, but it can mean that you're lacking fruits, vegetables, fiber, and micronutrients, which are all key components to optimizing your health while taking GLP-1 medications.

Here's a game plan for balancing your carbohydrate intake while still enjoying your favorite foods that may be more processed. The first part of the plan is to ensure with every meal you have a fruit or vegetable and ideally a whole-grain carbohydrate source (like whole-grain pasta, rice, tortillas, oats, etc.). This sets you up to be taking in the majority of your carbohydrates from fruits, vegetables, and whole grains. Ideally, you'll want to follow step one for at least 80 percent of the meals you eat in a week. If you eat three meals a day, that means you'd want about seventeen of your weekly meals to follow step one.

Then the second part is to allow the other roughly 20 percent of your meals (about four per week) to include more of those processed carbohydrates that you can have in your healthy food intake in moderation.

As you are human, there's always going to be a degree of flexibility you should allow when trying to balance out your carbohydrate intake. If you have a few extra days here or there where your 80 to 20 ratio is slightly off, don't sweat it; keep moving forward!

72 Simplify Your Starches

Here's a quick fact for you: Not all carbohydrates are starches. There's a lot of misconceptions around starches and rhetoric that starches are bad for you and should be avoided. However, that's simply not true. Some of the most common starches you eat are packed with great micronutrients and fiber, which are critical for your health. There are, however, foods that are highly processed that do have a high starch content. So when you think about starches in your diet, to get the micronutrient and fiber benefits you want, aim for foods that haven't been highly processed.

To simplify getting your starches in throughout the day, start by creating a list on paper or on your phone, or make a mental list of your favorite starches. Starch can be found in easily accessible foods like potatoes, corn, rice, whole-grain breads, cereals, pasta, oats, and legumes. Plantains are a bit less common but also a great starch source packed with vitamins C and A, and potassium too. Once you have your list of starches you enjoy, try to keep a stash of different starch sources in your pantry or refrigerator. Aim to have at least one serving of starches at each of your meals. This helps get not only general calories in you but more specifically supports your carbohydrate intake, which is key for energy. Starches are important for digestive health, staying satiated, and for energy levels; the latter, especially, is important when taking a GLP-1 medication because low energy and fatigue are very common.

73 Vary Your Vegetables

Vegetable intake can be the bane of some people's existence, but it doesn't have to be. You may be thinking "I eat vegetables; I'm sure I am fine," which may be true if you are having at least four to five servings of vegetables per day. If you want to have optimal health while taking a GLP-1 medication, it's not just the act of eating vegetables that matters, it's also the variety. Creating variety in your vegetable intake is important because it allows for a greater mix of micronutrients and allows for the healthy bacteria in your microbiome to have a variety of food sources to support healthy levels.

It's no secret that vegetables are a great source of fiber (which is key for regular bowel movements, a healthy microbiome, and cholesterol levels) and micronutrients, but what's less talked about is how important the variety of your vegetables is. If you're someone who is barely getting enough vegetables as is, you'll want to focus on just eating your vegetables until it's a consistent habit. On the flip side, if you're wanting to optimize your GLP-1 journey and are already eating the minimum number of vegetables that is recommended, try taking your vegetable intake to the next level by focusing on a variety of vegetables every week.

A seamless way to keep a rotation of vegetables flowing, without creating too much hassle for you, would be to lean on seasonal vegetables. By picking vegetables that are in season, you have a change of vegetables every few months to choose from. Try to incorporate at least five types of vegetables throughout the week, then the following week try to replace two or three of those five vegetables with a different kind.

74 | Have Fun with Fruits

If you're struggling with getting enough fruit into your meal plans, like so many do, try changing how you look at fruit intake. When you think about getting enough servings of fruit each day, you may default to thinking of picking up a piece of fruit and eating it, but there's more to life than that; you can actually make hitting your fruit intake goals fun!

Here are a few ways to add some variety to your fruit choices:

- **Create a new favorite smoothie.** Pack a smoothie with your favorite fruit blend. Try a berry assortment of blackberries, raspberries, and strawberries, or strawberry and banana, or mango and pineapple; the possibilities are endless!

- **Crack open canned fruit.** This can be a great option if you are trying to be more budget conscious or are on the go. Aim for the canned fruit that has no sugar added. You can create a quick and fun fruit salad for variety!

- **Stock your freezer with fruit.** Frozen fruit is just as great as fresh fruit and you don't have to worry about it going bad before you can eat it. The best part about frozen fruit? It allows you to have out-of-season fruits like cherries or mangoes during the colder months, no waiting until summer!

Throughout the day aim to have at least three fruits, if not more; that ensures you're getting great fiber intake and the micronutrients you need.

75 Include In-Season Fruits

It's true that with the world of frozen fruits and vegetables available, you don't technically ever have to go without most fruits since you can always find them in the frozen section. However, there are health benefits to eating the fruits that are in season if you're able to (a bonus financial benefit is that in some cases seasonal produce can be less expensive).

In-season fruits typically have higher levels of vitamins and minerals and can pack an extra antioxidant punch. They also typically are fresher and have a stronger flavor profile, which can be tastier and more enjoyable. You're also more likely to incorporate more natural variety in your fruit intake by focusing on eating fruits that are currently in season, which can be beneficial for your microbiome. When taking a GLP-1 medication, the more variety you have in your fruit intake, the better for digestion, and the more variety, the more likely you are to consume all the micronutrients you need. Here's a list of what's in season when, to help you easily incorporate seasonal fruit into your food intake:

- **Spring:** apples, bananas, avocados, kiwis, apricots, pineapple, strawberries
- **Summer:** apples, bananas, apricots, blackberries, blueberries, cherries, cantaloupe, honeydew melon, watermelon, peaches, plums, raspberries, strawberries, mangoes
- **Fall:** apples, bananas, cranberries, kiwis, mangoes, pears, raspberries, pineapple
- **Winter:** apples, avocados, bananas, kiwis, grapefruits, oranges, pomegranates, pears

76 Get Clear on Carbohydrates

Carbohydrates are an essential part of a well-rounded diet. Unfortunately in this day and age of social media they have become a villain in the story of many, but unfairly so. It's important to remember that when taking GLP-1 medications carbohydrates are necessary to help stabilize your blood sugar levels and avoid low blood sugar episodes. They also directly support you with symptom relief when taking GLP-1s. The fiber from carbohydrates helps regulate bowel movements, plus the bland foods that are encouraged if you're feeling ill are primarily all carbohydrates (they are stomach-settling champions).

Carbohydrates are also:

- Your body's preferred source of fuel
- Critical for brain and hormone function
- Important for fiber intake
- Delicious (this one maybe snuck itself in here, but it's not wrong!)

Now that you know how beneficial carbohydrates are, you can keep two considerations in mind on your GLP-1 journey:

- Carbohydrates should account for 45–65 percent of your overall calorie intake each day.
- Aim to pair your carbohydrates with a protein or fat at all your meals for blood sugar response support.

77 Find the Right Fats

When you're taking a GLP-1 medication, the quality of your food intake, especially your fat intake, is more important than ever. This stems from the fact that GLP-1 medications typically lead to a decrease in overall food intake and a decreased tolerance of fatty foods. So finding the right fats for your diet is important for your overall optimal nutrient intake but also to help avoid side effects.

The first step toward finding the right fats is knowing what kind of fats to avoid. Primarily you'll want to avoid fried foods and foods (and meals) that are extremely high in fat (consuming too many fats in one sitting can cause you to become ill). The second step is to take a mental inventory of what fat sources you already are consuming regularly: Are they primarily coming from meat sources or dairy products (red meats, butter, cheese, full-fat dairy) or are they coming from nuts, seeds, avocados, and olives?

If you are consuming more saturated fats (red meats, butter, and so on), your third step will be to slowly decrease the serving sizes of those saturated fats and eventually swap them for unsaturated fats. If you are already getting most of your fat intake from unsaturated fats, you'll want to adjust how many grams of fats you're eating at each setting. Pay attention to whether you're cooking with fats as well; if you are cooking with fats like olive oil and then including other fats as part of your meal (olives, avocados, nuts, and so on), it can quickly become more fat than you can tolerate at once. Last tip for finding your right fats: Utilize cooking oil sprays instead of free-flowing oil to better control your portion size.

78 Delay Digestion with Fat Intake

Believe it or not, your fat intake can actually impact your digestion. When fats are being digested, cholecystokinin secretion is stimulated; this hormone signals to your body to delay gastric emptying. Gastric emptying may sound familiar since you are taking a GLP-1 medication and one of the many functions of a GLP-1 medication is to delay gastric emptying. This is important to understand because you can manipulate your fat intake to work with you rather than potentially allowing it to make you sick. (A quick reminder: If food sits in your stomach for too long, chances are you are probably going to be sick to get the food out of your stomach.)

When gastric emptying is slowed from a combination of fat intake and your GLP-1 medication, this helps you stay fuller longer. This can be a benefit if you are someone who finds you are hungry frequently. To use fats to your advantage to help curb hunger further, you'll want to be smart about your fat intake.

The best way to do this is to focus on solid sources of fat rather than liquid fats. Solid sources would include healthy options like nuts, seeds, avocados, fish, and olives. Incorporate at least one serving of a healthy fat source at each of your meals or snacks to get the benefit of slower gastric emptying to keep you feeling fuller longer. Ensure that you are not taking in too much fat at once as that can increase your odds of digestive distress while taking a GLP-1 medication. You should aim to keep your fat intake at around 10–15 grams per meal. (Some people may have a higher fat tolerance; you can experiment to determine what's best for you.) Be sure to also use caution when adding fats to help ensure you're not overdoing your saturated fat intake in the process.

79 Watch the Types of Fats You Eat

If you think back to your high school science class, you may remember learning about bonds that hold molecules together. If you don't remember, that's okay; here's a quick crash course on how this topic relates to dietary fats. Saturated fats contain single bonds between carbon molecules while unsaturated fats contain double bonds. This creates a difference in structure; typically saturated fats are more solid at room temperature. Common saturated fats include butter, coconut oil, red meat, heavy cream, and cheese.

Unsaturated fats can be looked at in two smaller categories: polyunsaturated (which have multiple double bonds) and monounsaturated (which have one double bond). Unsaturated fats are found in olives, nuts, avocados, sunflower seeds, fish, flaxseed, and several oils (olive, flax, safflower, and soybean). Ideally you want the majority of your daily fat intake to come from unsaturated fats as they're more health protective than saturated fats.

Excessive fat intake can lead to unwelcome health problems like high cholesterol, obesity, and heart disease, so it's important to eat the right amount of the healthier fats without overdoing it. To help keep your saturated fat intake on the lower side try to:

- Pick reduced-fat or low-fat options when available.
- Focus on eating leaner cuts of meat with lower fat content.
- Measure out butter when using it to avoid overconsuming.
- Use alternatives to butter like olive oil spreads.
- Limit red meat consumption to one or two times per week.

Remember, moderation and balance is key. If you are someone who currently eats a diet high in saturated fats, focus on making small changes one at a time.

80 Calculate Your Specific Macronutrient Needs

If you want to be as specific and efficient as possible with your food tracking, tracking your macronutrients (or macros for short) can be a great tool to implement regularly. On your GLP-1 journey, tracking can be a great educational tool to understand the individual calorie, protein, carbohydrate, and fat content of different foods and their correlating serving sizes. If this is the route you'd like to take, you can either outsource your calculation to a dietitian or you can calculate your macro targets yourself.

To calculate your macronutrient needs you will:

1 **Start with your overall maintenance calories.** Use your total daily energy expenditure (TDEE) or your calorie deficit target, whichever is applicable to you; this will be your calorie target.

2 **Calculate your protein target.** To do this, pick 20–25 percent of your daily calorie target; this will be your calories from protein. Take that number and divide it by 4 (4 calories per 1 gram of protein); this equals the number of grams for your daily protein target.

3 **Calculate your fat target.** Pick 20–30 percent of your calorie target (30 percent if you're at maintenance, roughly 20–25 percent if in a deficit). Take that number and divide it by 9 (9 calories per 1 gram of fat); this equals the number of grams for your daily fat target.

4 **Calculate your carbohydrate target.** Take the calories that are left from your overall calorie target (this should be 45–60 percent of your overall daily intake) and divide that number by 4 (4 calories per 1 gram of carbohydrate); this equals the number of grams for your daily carbohydrate target.

This gives you general macronutrient targets that you can work on dialing in on to optimize your nutrition.

81 Tackling Food Tracking

For most people taking a GLP-1 medication, having some sort of oversight on their food intake, whether that's with specific calorie targets or macronutrient tracking, is beneficial because food intake can often drop too low. A decrease in appetite and changes to hunger signaling can lead to insufficient eating, so tracking your food intake can be helpful to ensure you're getting enough food overall and that you're getting enough of each macronutrient and micronutrient.

To track your food intake accurately you will want to get a food scale for the most accurate weighing of your foods. Measuring cups can also be helpful to get accurate readings on liquid items. Start with measuring out the amount that you are going to eat. Then you will need to input this information into a tracking app of your choice. There are many different tracking apps for you to pick from; find one that fits your preferences and budget (they range from free to annual paid subscriptions). Once you enter your food into the tracking app for each meal and snack, you will be able to see your calorie total and total grams of protein, carbohydrates, fats, fiber, and micronutrients as well.

This allows you to either track to a specific calorie goal or track to a range for calories, macronutrients, or other inputs. You'll also be able to pinpoint any possible issues with your nutrient intake with food tracking to help avoid or resolve any side effects like fatigue, nausea, or hair loss quickly. While it may not be for everyone, tracking may be for you if you're willing to try!

82 Try Alternative Food-Tracking Methods

Whether you have had a negative experience with tracking your calories or macronutrients before and don't want to track that closely, or you simply don't feel like it's right for you but still want a way to monitor your food intake, you're in luck as there are multiple ways to keep an eye on your food consumption. Two popular alternatives to tracking are the plate method and estimating your portion sizes by comparing them to objects or your hand size (see the following two entries).

You can find the best alternative tracking method for you by trying them each for two to four weeks to see if they work in your daily life or not. It's also important to consider that during different times in your life you may need to swap to a different method of food tracking to better accommodate your lifestyle. For example, if you are regularly on the go and relying on more liquid meals like smoothies or soups, the plate method likely wouldn't be your best fit. Instead, you could use portion size estimates while you're making your smoothie or soup so you have a better idea of your nutritional intake.

To give yourself your best chance of success with an alternative method of food tracking, think through your daily time, your lifestyle and environment, and if you feel any preference toward one method over the other. Once you've thought it through, give it your best shot for a few weeks and note how you're feeling as you get into a routine with it.

83 Adjust the Plate Method for GLP-1 Eating

The plate method is a common alternative to tracking that relies more on your accurate serving sizes portioned out by sections on your plate. The goal behind the plate method is to encourage enough fruit and vegetable intake, adequate protein intake, and to moderate carbohydrate intake. While taking your GLP-1 medication, the plate method can be a great way to keep tabs on your food intake without tracking every single ingredient you eat, but it's worth noting that while taking your GLP-1 you may need to utilize a modified version of the plate method.

The traditional plate method guidelines allow for half your plate to be non-starchy vegetables, a quarter of your plate as protein, and a quarter of your plate carbohydrates, plus a few tablespoons of fats. The traditional plate method also allows for fruit to be added to meals as well. When on your GLP-1 medication you can adapt the plate method to meet your needs by:

- Adjusting the overall size of your plate to be smaller to accommodate for smaller and more frequent meals.
- Allowing your half plate of vegetables to be a regular combination of fruits and vegetables rather than just vegetables.
- Slightly increasing the protein section of your plate to allow for a bit more protein intake.

If you're going to give the plate method a try, keep in mind that you don't want to have any giant piles of food on your plate, as this would put you over the section on your plate. This approach can be a great alternative to manage carbohydrate intake and increase protein intake, which can be two common areas that need adjusting when on your GLP-1.

84 Use Portion Size Estimates

Estimating your portion sizes for your meals and snacks can be a great way to control your individual meal intake and overall calorie intake without having to track anything individually. You may find that with portion size estimations it takes away stress with eating out or eating meals that have been made for you. Portion size estimates also allow for more flexibility in your food intake, which can help foster a positive relationship with monitoring your food intake. You can estimate your portions by comparing them to parts of your hand or common objects.

- Your hand when it makes a fist or the size of a baseball is roughly 1 cup (can be used for roughly a serving of vegetables or fruits).
- The palm of your hand or a deck of cards is roughly 3 ounces of meat (can be used for fish, poultry, red meats).
- Your thumb is roughly 1 tablespoon (can be used for spreads like almond butter).
- The tip of your finger or a postage stamp is roughly 1 teaspoon (can be used to portion out oils and fats).
- A scooped handful or a tennis ball is roughly 1/2 cup (can be used to portion out 1 ounce of grains).

If you want to try portion size estimates, aim to build your meals with at least one of each part of your hand or one object to create a well-rounded meal. The process will get easier the more you practice it.

85   Meal Plan Like a Pro

Meal planning isn't for everyone, but if you want to give it a try, you have a few options to make it as helpful as possible. If you're following a meal plan, you don't necessarily need to use a tracking app if you already know the nutritional content of the meals you're eating; a meal plan can be nice if you need more structure and don't have a ton of extra daily time to track in an app. Meal plans can be restrictive and have the potential to create disordered eating patterns if you're not using them safely. The key is to utilize meal planning to create a weekly plan that still has flexibility so you can use it as a foundation and adjust as needed.

You can sign up for sites where you enter your personal nutrition information and they give you entire weeks of eating plans paired with a grocery list of what you'll need to cook those meals. You can also work with a dietitian to get a customized meal plan to meet your specific needs and preferences. However, if you want to meal plan like a pro on your own, you can do it yourself with a little time. To plan out your own meals for the week, start by taking it one meal at a time. Plan your breakfasts, then lunches, dinners, and don't forget your snacks. Utilize the benefit of leftovers for lunch or even repeat dinners. You want to make it as easy as possible for yourself while also maintaining enough variety. Don't forget your fruit and vegetable intake goals while you're making your plan!

86　Build Your GLP-1 Grocery List

Your newest weekly nutrition habit is making your grocery list! While technically you can stroll into the grocery store and grab what looks or sounds good, you'll thank yourself later if you put a few minutes and a bit of intention behind your grocery list. When you're shopping without a plan, you're more likely to have gaps in your nutrition, and when taking a GLP-1 medication, you don't want to leave any gaps. With just a few minutes each week, you can use a three-step grocery plan to ensure you have well-balanced meals and snacks that are ready to fuel your GLP-1 journey.

STEP ONE

Create your master list. This can be a spreadsheet, paper list, or digital list. Include all the things you like in each of these categories: meats and fish, dairy products, nuts, seeds, fruits, vegetables, grains, condiments, canned items, and premade snacks. List all the foods you enjoy in each category (example: meats—chicken, ground turkey, salmon, shrimp, pork).

STEP TWO

Create your meal pairings for a balanced snack or meal. Ideally every meal or snack should include a protein source, a carbohydrate, and a fat (most of the time). You'll want to grab from your master list to create five to ten combinations for breakfast, lunch, dinner, and snacks to give yourself variety. Don't forget to include your favorite sauces or condiments to add flavor and variety. You can redo step two as many times as you'd like to maximize your number of combinations.

STEP THREE

Take a weekly planner and tentatively add in your daily meals.

When you know what you want to eat each day, you can take your plan to the grocery store to grab everything you need to have a nutritious week of meals.

87 Read Those Nutrition Labels

It's important to be able to understand and know how to decipher nutrition labels to be able to make the most informed decisions for your food choices and goals. Specifically, while you are on a GLP-1 medication, understanding nutrition labels is key so you're able to pick out products that support your goals pertaining to proteins, fats, fiber-rich foods, and overall calorie intake.

When looking at an entire nutrition label there is a plethora of information, so for the sake of simplicity on your GLP-1 journey look specifically at: grams of protein, grams of total fat and saturated fat, grams of fiber, and total calories (all relative to the serving size). Focusing on these four areas allows you to make informed decisions about your food intake without requiring too much extra work or brainpower.

As you know, protein intake is important on your GLP-1 journey to support your muscle mass and energy levels, and to combat side effects. Total fat is important to monitor overall to ensure you're getting the necessary dietary fat needed daily without overdoing it, while also making sure that you're not consuming too many saturated fats. Fiber is a key component to managing blood sugar levels and healthy bowel movements. Calorie intake should be monitored at a minimum every few weeks to ensure your food intake is not dropping too low.

Whether you check every nutrition label you come across or just do occasional checks to be certain you're getting enough of what you need, it's a powerful tool in your GLP-1 journey.

88 Implement the Mediterranean Diet

While incorporating a strict diet or meal plan may work for some people, it likely won't be long term and sustainable for most people. However, you may be a person who prefers to have more structure with your eating; if so, it might be beneficial to try the Mediterranean diet.

The Mediterranean diet is more of a framework for eating rather than a traditional diet that you may be thinking of. In terms of your GLP-1 journey, it can be followed when you're at maintenance, if you're in a deficit, or even if you're in a surplus. The main components of the Mediterranean diet are fruits and vegetables, lean protein sources, whole grains, healthy fats, nuts and legumes, some dairy, and limited red meat.

To start implementing the Mediterranean diet into each of your meals, look at your fruits and vegetables first. Ensure you include a fruit and vegetable ideally with every meal and snack throughout the day. Then focus on your fat sources: Swap out your fat sources for olive oil and add in nuts, seeds, and olives to your daily intake. When you are planning your protein, pick lean protein sources such as poultry as your main protein, add fish two to three times per week, and limit red meat to one to two times per week. Grains should be from whole-grain sources like whole-grain pasta, couscous, or quinoa to name a few. You'll want to make these the staples of your meals, and limit processed foods like pastries, sweets, white breads, juice, soda, and alcohol.

89 Pass on the Fasting

There are several methods of fasting that have become popular, but most are versions of intermittent fasting, and when you're on your GLP-1 journey this is one of the last approaches you should be taking to have a successful experience. When you are taking a GLP-1 medication, your digestion is slowed through delayed gastric emptying and slowed motility through your gastrointestinal tract. Fasting for long periods of time can also decrease motility, which then can compound the effects of your GLP-1 medication and lead to constipation, bloating, or other discomforts with meals, the result being that you're not able to get all your necessary food intake in. Since you feel fuller faster and for longer on GLP-1 medications, you cannot rely on larger, less frequent meals without falling short on your food intake or making yourself sick.

It's also possible that when combining fasting with GLP-1 medications that are working to improve your insulin and blood sugar regulation and response, you could be leading yourself to more instances of low blood sugar levels. When your blood sugar drops, your body will naturally try to correct it and bring it up. If this cycle becomes a regular pattern from regular fasting, it can worsen blood sugar control and worsen your health outcomes, which is exactly what you may be taking a GLP-1 to avoid.

Rather than fasting, build a regular meal schedule to support you while taking your GLP-1 medication. When you have breakfast within an hour of waking up (with 20–30 grams of protein), then a balanced meal or snack roughly every 3–4 hours after breakfast, you set yourself up for stable blood sugar levels, and you'll be able to get your food intake in more easily.

90 | Avoid the Keto Conundrum

While the keto diet originated with the purpose of supporting the epileptic population for seizure reduction, there's been an increase in recent years of using the keto diet for dieting purposes. The keto diet is focused on low carbohydrate (only 20–50 grams per day) and high fat intake to force the body to rely on ketones instead of glucose. It is often not executed correctly and people are not in actual ketosis, which then results in eating fewer carbohydrates; this translates to a low intake of fruits, vegetables, fiber, and micronutrients and a high intake of fats (often with increased saturated fat intake), which is not ideal for overall health. For most people, a keto diet also is not a realistic way of eating for long periods and thus isn't sustainable.

In addition, your GLP-1 journey and the keto diet do not pair well together. Not only is it not indicated for use with GLP-1 medications, but the keto diet also has major nutritional gaps that directly contradict best practices when on GLP-1s. Keto's emphasis on fats can quickly make you sick because fats slow digestion and digestive distress can follow high fat intake on GLP-1s. And fiber intake from carbohydrates, which is lacking in a keto diet, is key to managing fatigue, hair loss, nausea, and other side effects while taking your GLP-1.

While the keto diet may seem alluring or like a quick way to expedite results, long term it's not likely to give you success with your health outcomes. Instead of removing the majority of your carbohydrates to follow the keto diet, focus on the quality of your carbohydrate intake to feel energized, stay satisfied, and keep your blood work in check.

91 Get Your Must-Have Supplements

Supplementation should complement a well-rounded diet to be most effective; however, supplements can also be helpful in specific cases to help bridge any potential gaps in your dietary intake. When you start your GLP-1 medication or have a dose increase, you may experience more instances of side effects or changes to your food intake as you adjust the foods you are eating. When this happens, it can create nutrient gaps, whether from not getting enough of the food itself due to learning new eating habits or from side effects like nausea preventing you from eating and drinking.

To bridge this gap, you can have three staple supplements on deck for your GLP-1 journey: a high-quality multivitamin, a protein powder, and electrolytes. These three items can create a well-rounded supplement routine to help keep you on track and minimize symptoms. A multivitamin is key to support those vitamin and mineral gaps that can be present from insufficient calorie intake or insufficient fruit and vegetable intake. Protein powder can add easy protein with minimal volume or effort. Electrolytes can help with increasing water intake and be a constipation fighter when paired with adequate water and fiber intake.

There are hundreds of supplements on the market, so how can you safely build your must-have supplement stack? Look for third-party tested supplements for safety, research the brand that you are interested in to ensure they are a legitimate company, and also understand that all supplements are not created equal: If it seems too good to be true, it probably is!

92 Investigate Your Multivitamin

Multivitamins are numerous in the supplement market, and although experts continue to debate the benefits they provide for the general population, if you're taking a GLP-1 you should consider a multivitamin. Of course, not any multivitamin will do for you on your GLP-1 journey, and it's important to understand that supplements vary widely in quality. Supplements are largely not regulated and with that can come increased risk for possible contaminants or falsified or inaccurate ingredient claims. When you are taking a GLP-1 medication that can lead to possible nutrient deficiencies, a multivitamin can help bridge the gap while you work on optimizing your food intake. This can help prevent hair loss, improve or prevent fatigue, and help you feel your best.

When you are searching for a multivitamin, one way to get peace of mind about the product's quality is to find out if it is NSF Certified for Sport. This designation means there are no prohibited substances or masking agents, and the ingredients in the product are what they claim to be, which is important for athletes or anyone who could be tested for banned substances. Even if you are not an elite athlete, you want to know that your vitamins and supplements are what they say they are. Thorne is a great option for multivitamins that are NSF Certified for Sport. For any products you are considering, confirm with the company via their website or customer service that they third-party test their supplements to check that there are not any harmful contaminants and that their product contains the correct amounts that they claim they have. Lastly, make sure your multivitamin includes at least magnesium, potassium, vitamin D, and calcium. Thorne, Pure Encapsulations, and Ritual are great choices for multivitamins.

93 Stay Balanced with Electrolytes

Electrolytes such as sodium, potassium, magnesium, and calcium are essential minerals your body needs to function properly every day. You typically get enough calcium from your food intake, but sodium, potassium, and magnesium are a trio that's best added as a supplement in conjunction with dietary intake, especially while taking your GLP-1 medication.

Electrolytes are the solution for a whole host of issues, like:

- **Low energy levels and fatigue:** Electrolytes directly impact your energy levels to give you that much-needed boost.
- **Rapid weight loss:** If you're a hyper-responder who drops weight quickly on GLP-1s, those rapid weight loss changes impact your fluid and electrolyte balance. Avoid issues like dizziness, lightheadedness, and even fainting by using electrolytes to balance things out.
- **Constipation:** Regular electrolyte use each day can help keep your bowels moving and keep constipation at bay.
- **Diarrhea:** If you are someone who struggles with diarrhea, you're constantly losing electrolytes and it's critical to replenish them to stay balanced.

The trio of sodium, magnesium, and potassium together can be found in high-quality electrolyte supplements that you can grab online or at your local store.

94 **Power Up with Protein Powders**

Supplemental protein intake can be incredibly helpful to have in your daily routine while taking a GLP-1 medication. Sufficient protein is key to managing nausea, preventing unnecessary muscle mass loss, preventing hair loss, preventing or improving fatigue, and supporting healthy blood sugar regulation, among other benefits. When you don't eat enough protein, your body will break down your muscle for the amino acids it needs. Unfortunately, when you take your GLP-1 medication you may experience aversions to proteins (most commonly meats) for short periods of time. This can make it difficult to consume enough protein each day to support your health and keep side effects away.

Protein powders or premade protein shakes can be great options to add once a day to give you a baseline 20–30 grams of protein without having to eat a whole meal with more volume. For most protein powders, you can combine them with as little as 8 ounces of water or your milk of choice to get the entire serving of protein. The ability to consume a lower volume of food with a higher protein content is especially helpful if you are finding that you're becoming full quickly or are experiencing nausea. Starting your day with a protein shake, either homemade or premade, can help you quickly get sustenance in you—which can cure early morning nausea without much effort.

Thorne, Naked Nutrition, Owyn, Clean Simple Eats, and 1Up Nutrition are all third-party–tested protein powder or premade protein shake brands that have whey protein and plant protein options that can provide great supplemental protein.

95 | Keep Away from GLP-1 Supplements

The last thing you need is to fall victim to a scam and that's exactly what those GLP-1 supplements that are being marketed to you are. These so-called GLP-1 supplements aren't regular supplements like a multivitamin, electrolytes, or protein powder; these are supplements that are claiming to naturally increase your own GLP-1 production or boost your results on your GLP-1 medication. These supplements have great marketing behind them and that's about it.

Here's the skinny on these GLP-1–boosting supplements: The claims they make don't have evidence to back them up and you should save your money and avoid them. Utilize your money and resources on building out a robust dietary intake with fruits, vegetables, protein, whole grains, and healthy fats. Focus on strength training, adequate rest, staying hydrated, and managing your stress. Together, this will take you further than any supplement that's marketed to boost your natural GLP-1 intake. What they call "nature's Ozempic" is also known as berberine, but it is not legitimate. Berberine is a completely separate supplement that can have some benefits but it's not comparable to a GLP-1 injectable medication. Remember that in the world of social media, most things are too good to be true. You should always check with a healthcare provider on the legitimacy of claims you see online, especially with nutrition or health products.

96 Say Good Riddance to Greens Powders

Greens powders: They're all the rage, they're marketed well, the branding is eye-catching, influencers are selling you on them, and they're on the shelves at numerous stores. If you're a hardcore greens powder lover, you can continue to use them; they're not going to be stripped away from you. However, a common question among people taking GLP-1 medications is "should you take a greens powder supplement?" and the answer is no.

Taking a greens powder supplement is in no way a requirement to see success while taking a GLP-1 medication and there's also not enough evidence to prove that greens powders have any benefit. The main point of your fruit and vegetable intake is to consume the micronutrients and fiber found in them, and when you grind the fruits and vegetables into a dry powder, you're going to lose some of the nutrients and also lose the fiber content. When taking a GLP-1 medication, a major player in managing side effects is fiber intake, and greens powders will not assist in this.

At the end of the day, the best advice is to save yourself the money, skip the greens powders, and direct your attention to a great multivitamin paired with enough fruits and vegetables in your diet. If you'd like to continue on your greens powder journey, just be sure they are third-party tested so you don't accidentally eat heavy metals (which are commonly found in greens powders).

97 Focus On Pre- and Post-Workout Nutrition

Regular exercise, whether it's individual resistance training, group fitness classes, or personal training sessions, can be beneficial to your GLP-1 journey, and you should focus on your nutrition before and after your workouts to create a better workout experience and outcome. By dialing in your pre- and post-workout nutrition, you're able to maximize your energy during your workouts, support muscle growth and recovery, and improve your athletic performance when you are properly fueled.

Your nutrition habits before your workout can have a major influence on your ability to push through harder workouts and progress with your workouts, whether strength related or endurance related. Even if you're an early riser who enjoys an early morning workout, you should ideally still be having breakfast roughly an hour before your workout. Throughout the rest of the day, if you are planning to work out you'll want to aim to:

- Have a pre-workout meal or snack: If it's a meal it should be 3–4 hours before exercise, whereas a snack can be 1–3 hours before exercise.
- Have at least 16–24 ounces of water in the 2–3 hours leading up to your exercise session.

After your workout, to ensure that you're set up to recover, repair your muscle tissue, replenish lost fluids, and recharge, you'll want to aim to:

- Replenish fluids via water intake or sports drinks or electrolytes.
- Have a post-workout meal focused on protein and carbohydrates within 2 hours of your workout, ideally sooner rather than later.

When you're seeing improvements in performance and energy, and are recovering more quickly, you can thank yourself for focusing on your pre- and post-workout nutrition.

98 Get the Lowdown on Fiber

Dietary fiber comes from carbohydrates and has two forms: soluble fiber and insoluble fiber. Overall, fiber is responsible for supporting healthy bowels, healthy bowel movements, and healthy cholesterol levels, and it improves blood sugar levels and even impacts satiety when eating.

When you are taking a GLP-1 medication and want to avoid the common side effect of constipation, one of the foundational things you should do is ensure that there's enough fiber in your daily intake. As the average daily dietary intake for most people is deficient in fruits, vegetables, and whole grains, it also correlates that their fiber intake is also typically too low. When you have enough fiber in your diet each day, paired with adequate water intake, you'll be able to prevent most constipation that can come with GLP-1 medications and you'll also be contributing to improving your other health metrics like blood sugar and cholesterol. Foods that are good sources of fiber are also usually more filling, which helps with your satiety (aka keeping you feeling fuller longer).

But how do you know how much fiber is enough? Here are the minimum values:

- **Women under 50 years old:** at least 25 grams per day
- **Women over 50 years old:** at least 21 grams per day
- **Men under 50 years old:** at least 38 grams per day
- **Men over 50 years old:** at least 30 grams per day

If you're lacking in the fiber intake department, increase in small amounts of 2–3 grams per day to avoid causing constipation with increased fiber intake. Your body will adapt to the recommended daily amount with consistency.

99   Know the Benefits of Soluble Fiber

Soluble fiber is fiber that supports healthy cholesterol levels and blood sugar regulation. When mixed with water in your body, soluble fiber becomes a gel-like consistency and as it slowly moves through the body it slows down your digestion. Since your digestion is slowed down, this allows food to be broken down more slowly and absorbed at a slower rate. This creates a lower rise in glucose levels after meals, which can support a healthy blood sugar response. Soluble fiber also can bind to cholesterol and remove it from your body rather than letting it enter the bloodstream, so it can have a profound effect on managing healthy cholesterol levels as well.

You'll find soluble fiber in fruits, vegetables, grains, nuts, and seeds. The concentration of soluble fiber per serving size varies depending on the food itself, but if you keep a steady rotation of fruits, vegetables, nuts, grains, and seeds in your daily intake you shouldn't have to do anything extravagant to meet your needs. Fruit sources with good amounts of soluble fiber include figs, pears, avocados, apricots, apples, nectarines, and guava. You can reach for flaxseed, sunflower seeds, hazelnuts, oats, or barley for soluble fiber. You can also bring in Brussels sprouts, turnips, carrots, sweet potatoes, and broccoli to your meals for easy soluble fiber.

While the exact amount of soluble fiber out of your total fiber intake doesn't have a set recommended amount, try to incorporate at least 10 grams of soluble fiber in your diet every day. You can get this amount by having ¾ cup of black beans and 1 cup of Brussels sprouts in one day.

100 Ingest More Insoluble Fiber

Insoluble fiber is responsible for adding bulk to your stools and helping keep digestion moving because it doesn't dissolve in water. This type of fiber is ideal for helping prevent constipation as it adds structure to the stool and helps keep your stool moving. It also pulls water into your intestines to keep your stool softer, which makes it easier to pass when you have a bowel movement.

While insoluble fiber is found in the same main food categories as soluble fiber (fruits, vegetables, nuts, seeds, whole grains), the individual sources can vary. You can incorporate insoluble fiber through vegetables like artichokes, kale, lima beans, potatoes with the skin on, edamame, sweet potatoes with skin on, raw carrots, and cooked Brussels sprouts. For fruits, berries like blueberries, strawberries, and raspberries are great options for insoluble fiber, plus mangoes, kiwis, apricots with the skin, red apples with skin, and pears. Raw almonds, walnuts, sesame seeds, sunflower seeds, flaxseed, cooked lentils, cooked kidney beans, cooked garbanzo beans, and cooked black beans can be quick additions to your day from the nuts, seeds, and beans categories. Last but not least, for grains try incorporating cooked brown rice, barley, oatmeal, quinoa, or whole-grain pasta, plus wheat bran to add to your insoluble fiber totals.

A quick rule for insoluble fiber is to aim to have about two-thirds of your overall fiber intake come from insoluble fiber sources, or for every 1 gram of soluble fiber, have 2 grams of insoluble fiber; either way, insoluble fiber should make up the majority of your daily fiber intake.

101 Don't Confuse Prebiotics and Probiotics

Prebiotics and probiotics are heavily marketed, but realistically you don't need a supplement to create a healthy, balanced intake of prebiotics and probiotics. While yes, they are found in supplement form, not all are created equal, or even absorbed from supplements to be effective. Instead, you should try intentional intake of prebiotic- and probiotic-rich foods to fulfill your needs.

When taking a GLP-1 medication, you know that your digestive system is directly impacted. Since your gastric emptying and motility is decreased while taking GLP-1s, that leads to food sitting in your digestive system longer than it would without a GLP-1 medication. Ensuring you get enough prebiotics and probiotics from your food intake can help maintain healthy levels of bacteria, otherwise known as a healthy microbiome. Maintaining a healthy, balanced microbiome helps strengthen your body's immune system, supports lower levels of inflammation, promotes weight loss, and helps with blood sugar regulation.

Prebiotics are foods that feed the healthy bacteria in your colon. They are found in foods that don't get broken down during the digestion process so that they can survive until they reach your colon, where they become food for your gut bacteria. Probiotics, on the other hand, are live microorganisms contained in some foods that support your digestive health and immune system. In an ideal world, you'll want to include a variety of prebiotic and probiotic sources in your food intake every day at each meal to support your microbiome during your GLP-1 journey.

102 Preplan Your Prebiotic Foods

Prebiotics are often forgotten because their close relative, probiotics, get so much attention, but they're also very important to your gut health. Without sufficient prebiotic intake, you'll not be able to experience the benefits of a healthy microbiome. Think of prebiotics and probiotics as salt and pepper: They are their own things, but they complement each other and are better together. Prebiotics are found in common foods that you should already be incorporating to support your fiber intake while taking a GLP-1 medication. Most prebiotic foods are also high in fiber, so your preplanning of your prebiotic foods can complement your preplanning of your fiber intake.

Common prebiotic-rich foods include garlic, onions, asparagus, bananas, avocados, apples, oats, flaxseed, barley, and cocoa. There's also jicama and yacon root, leeks, and Jerusalem artichokes that are not as common but still can be incorporated if you enjoy them. To have the highest prebiotic benefit from food sources, it's best to use them in their raw form as cooking can alter their structures.

There's no set recommendation for how many grams of prebiotics you should eat per day to keep your microbiome flourishing; however, incorporating at least 5 grams per day can be a baseline. If you currently don't have a regular variety of prebiotic-rich foods in your diet, you'll want to slowly work up to the 5 grams per day to avoid causing digestive issues like bloating or excessive gas production.

103 Unleash the Power of Probiotic Foods

Probiotics are a powerful part of your daily food intake to help you feel your best, but if you're not intentional about packing probiotic-rich foods into your day, you may end up shortchanging yourself and your microbiome. Probiotics don't have a recommended daily intake, so the amount you take in will largely depend on how you stay on top of your probiotic-rich foods in your daily intake.

Probiotic-rich foods include dairy products like yogurt and kefir, and fermented foods and drinks like kombucha, miso, kimchi, tempeh, sauerkraut, and pickles. If you want to incorporate pickles be sure they have been fermented, as some pickles are only made with vinegar, which won't give you the same probiotic benefit. While you can eat these foods by themselves daily or have a glass of kombucha each morning, you can also hide them in recipes.

You can incorporate yogurt into snack dips, as a substitute for mayonnaise, or in baking recipes, sauces, salad dressings, or smoothies. Kefir can be used for overnight-oats parfaits, pasta dishes, sauces, or dips. Fermented sources of probiotics can be used as garnishes in your favorite dishes, on snack plates, in breakfast scrambles, on sandwiches, or in salad. There's no right or wrong way to incorporate probiotic-rich foods; what's most important is that you do include them regularly in your daily meals to keep your microbiome happy while on your GLP-1.

104 Stay Hydrated

If there's one single habit that can cause, worsen, or prolong unwanted side effects like fatigue, worsening nausea, and constipation while taking a GLP-1 medication, it's insufficient water intake. When you're dehydrated, it can lead to decreased cognitive function, poorer blood sugar regulation, and feeling extremely lethargic. It's also a quick way to create severe constipation where you are so uncomfortable you may need to lean on laxative-type medications for relief, but even those won't work well if you're not hydrated.

When you think about your water intake, you'll want to see where your intake lands currently to determine if you need to increase or maintain your intake. At a minimum, without factoring in warmer times of the year and exercise, you should have about half your body weight in ounces of water per day. If you find that your water intake is significantly lower than it should be, focus on increasing the amount of water you drink by 5–10 ounces per week until you are up to your target. Keep in mind you will likely have to pee more frequently while increasing your water intake, but this will level out and regulate the more consistently you drink enough water.

To help get more water intake you can try:

- Adding flavor to your water
- Setting reminders on your phone to take a few sips
- Using a larger water bottle
- Using a water bottle or cup that has a straw

105 Add a Little Flavor Naturally

Staying hydrated while taking your GLP-1 medication will go a long way in helping you prevent several side effects. If you're someone who doesn't enjoy drinking water in general or doesn't enjoy the taste of water, adding a little bit of flavor to your drinks can go a long way in motivating you to drink more and increase your water intake. Of course, not every single ounce of water you drink needs to be flavored, but you can use it as an incentive to get through drinking your normal water and then have flavored water (or if it's a deal breaker, use flavored water all the way).

There are flavoring packets and liquids you can buy from the store that have the same flavor as your favorite treats and can be fine to add in, but if you are trying to avoid artificial flavoring or sweeteners, you can take a more natural approach to adding flavor.

The easiest way to add natural flavor to your water is with fruits and herbs. Limes and lemons freshly squeezed into your glass pack a big flavor punch. You can also add other combinations that have a bigger impact if they are infused into your water. Strawberries with basil, strawberries with mint, mint and lime, orange and lime, and cucumber and lemon are just a few possible combination ideas. The idea is you will essentially let the fruit and herbs soak in the water to infuse the flavor. You can do this in a regular jar or bottle, or you can make a bigger batch of water in a pitcher to have a supply of flavored water on hand.

106 Avoid Alcohol

Everyone reacts differently to alcohol intake, but for most people, drinking alcohol while taking their GLP-1 medication results in a higher incidence of ending up ill (sometimes violently ill), even if they've only consumed one or two drinks. This won't be your average alcohol-related illness either; this will be gastrointestinal illness like vomiting or uncontrollable diarrhea, stomach cramps, and abdominal pain, paired with nausea, chills, and then some hangover-like symptoms the following day.

Alcohol can worsen side effects from GLP-1 medications for many, like nausea, diarrhea, indigestion, or vomiting. If you're someone who has experienced being sick after drinking while on your GLP-1, you're probably thinking that it is an activity you'll opt out of moving forward. Truly, for overall health and longevity, the less alcohol intake you have, the better. Alcohol is a toxin and does increase your risk of harm to your body. The best advice for alcohol intake while on your GLP-1? Limit your alcohol consumption and if possible avoid it completely.

If you decide to consume alcoholic beverages, keep in mind the recommended daily limits: one drink per day for women, or two drinks per day for men. You'll want to drink in moderation and monitor how your body reacts to alcohol to make your most informed decision about whether or not alcohol intake is worth it for you.

107 Take Caution with Caffeine Intake

Caffeine lovers can rejoice: Being on a GLP-1 medication does not mean that you have to remove caffeine from your daily intake. But you do need to use it wisely to support your health, and not abuse it to manage side effects from your GLP-1 medication. Fatigue is a well-documented side effect of GLP-1 medications, and when you're tired, you gravitate toward a caffeinated beverage like coffee, tea, or energy drinks to feel a boost in your energy. While this isn't inherently a bad thing, it can quickly become a problem if you're not being mindful of your total caffeine intake. It's also important to understand in the context of your GLP-1 journey that caffeine may not be a solution for your fatigue; you may actually need to correct other pieces of your diet like hydration and calorie intake to get relief from fatigue.

Before reaching for caffeine to help with your fatigue, stop and check to see how much water you've had throughout the day so far. If you're not solidly on the way to drinking at least half your body weight in ounces, skip the caffeine and have some water. Then, check your food intake. If you haven't had enough overall calories, protein, or carbohydrates throughout the day, or if it's been more than 3 hours since you've had a snack or meal, skip the caffeine and go get some sustenance. Wait 30–60 minutes to allow your system to course correct and address your fatigue, then you can add in some caffeine if you want or need to. Be sure to keep your caffeine intake lower than the recommended maximum daily amount of 400 milligrams per day.

108 Get the Lowdown on Artificial Sweeteners

The subject of artificial sweeteners often seems to cause controversy and conflict for GLP-1 users. You're told not to have artificial sweeteners, but then you're also told that you can have them in moderation. When you're getting two different pieces of advice that contradict each other, how can you know which to follow?

The reality is at the end of the day you'll want to make a decision on artificial sweeteners that aligns best with your preferences. If you enjoy sweets or sodas, there are many options that are low-calorie or no-calorie swaps thanks to artificial sweeteners. While working to improve your blood sugar and insulin levels or working to lose weight, these substitutes can be better options to manage calorie intake while still enjoying the things you like. So they can help you maintain a healthy relationship with your body and food.

On the flip side, you may notice that if you are regularly consuming foods or beverages with artificial sweeteners, it can cause you to experience increased cravings and increased hunger. This leads to a struggle to control portion sizes and overall food intake, which can work against your weight loss goals, not to mention it can create strain on your relationship with food. Additionally, it's worth noting that some people are more sensitive to artificial sweeteners; you may find that when eating them you are bloating more often or developing irregular bowel movements. This won't be the case for everyone but it's something to keep an eye on.

No matter what your preference for artificial sweeteners is, there's individual nuance to your relationship and preferences with them, so make the choice to have them freely, limit them completely, or enjoy them in moderation based on what you're comfortable with.

109 Drop Your Added Sugar Intake

Added sugars are sugars that get added to food and beverages during processing. You can monitor your overall added sugar intake by checking the nutrition labels on the foods and beverages you are consuming. There is a separate line item that shows the amount of added sugars right under the listing for total sugars. Added sugars can come from syrups, honey, concentrated vegetable juice, concentrated fruit juice, table sugar, or sucrose and dextrose. Added sugars are not the same as sugar that is found naturally in fruits or vegetables.

The Standard American Diet is typically high in added sugars from beverages that have been sweetened, baked foods, sweets, or foods like dairy products that have had sugar added for sweetness. Overall, you want to keep added sugars under 10 percent of your daily calories, so if you have 2,000 calories per day, you don't want more than 200 calories to come from added sugars per day.

To create healthier habits to complement your GLP-1 medication, do an audit on your overall added sugar intake and work on bringing it down to no more than 10 percent of your daily calorie intake. If you don't want to track your intake that closely, you can still decrease your added sugar intake by using nutrition labels to make intentional choices and changes. If the nutrition label says the added sugar is 5 percent or less of the daily value, it's considered low for added sugars, whereas 20 percent or more is considered high. Aim to read all nutrition labels for the foods and beverages you consume and make sure to have the majority (80 percent or more) of your choices fall into the low added sugars category.

110 Enjoy Eating Out on GLP-1s

An integral part of many people's social and personal lives includes eating out at restaurants. If you are battling side effects from your GLP-1 medication or are finding you can't eat the same foods or portion sizes, eating at a restaurant can be a nerve-wracking experience. Depending on your experience, it may even deter you from enjoying meals out. Fortunately, eating out doesn't have to be a dreaded experience; you can eat out and enjoy yourself while on your GLP-1 medication.

To have success with eating out, here are some quick tips that will help you to enjoy yourself and make the best nutrition decisions for your comfort and health:

- Ask for your meal to be cooked with cooking spray rather than oil or butter.
- Add on a vegetable as a side if your meal doesn't come with one automatically.
- Ask for a to-go container when your meal comes so you can save some for later and keep your portion size smaller.
- Tackle your protein and vegetable first before moving on to your carbohydrate.
- Avoid drinking large amounts of liquid at your meals; take only small sips to conserve stomach space for your food.
- Minimize snacking on appetizers. If you want an appetizer, add more of your main dish to your to-go box for later.
- Share an entrée or appetizer with someone else if you don't want to take leftovers home.
- Avoid having alcoholic beverages before, during, or after your meal.

Most importantly, chew slowly, take your time eating, and enjoy yourself!

4 | Lifestyle Update

Your lifestyle may need an update to keep up with your GLP-1 medication journey if you want it to be as positive of an experience as possible. Whenever you want to better your health, but especially when trying to reduce inflammation or lose weight, making lifestyle changes to support improved sleep, improved physical activity, and reduced stress will be essential steps.

GLP-1 medications offer a unique opportunity for those who decide to take them to completely transform their life and their health. The normal routines and habits that have taken you to where you are today may not fit into a new normal that includes a GLP-1 medication. It's never been more important to be realistic about your habits, your goals, and your expectations as you embark on your GLP-1 journey.

This chapter will be your guide to learning how to be realistic with yourself, your timelines for progress, your goals, and your consistency. You'll learn how to adjust your behaviors around your meals to best suit taking a GLP-1 medication and the changes that come with it, and most importantly you'll learn how to go through your GLP-1 experience with more kindness and compassion for yourself and your body.

111 Track Those Injections for the Best Results

Following your healthcare provider's recommendations regarding injecting your medication is paramount to seeing success on your GLP-1. GLP-1 medications start working in your body after you inject them and typically last in your system for about a week (hence the reason they are weekly injections).

Over multiple consecutive weeks and months the medication helps your body systems take full advantage of your GLP-1 medication. You might start to see improvements in overall inflammation, improvements in your insulin resistance or blood sugar levels, and your cholesterol may even decrease. You could be steadily losing weight as well. Overall, the consecutive weeks of injecting paired with your hard work are paying off. But then, you stop injecting consistently and your injections become sporadic. You miss doses altogether or take your injection a few days late each time by accident. Your insulin levels begin to rise again, your inflammation increases, your fatigue returns, and your appetite starts to feel unpredictable.

Every once in a while, if you are late with or miss a dose, it likely won't break your progress. However, if your inconsistency starts adding up, you're not going to see the same positive results as you could be seeing with consistency.

Leave the inconsistency behind you and track your injections to ensure you're not missing your doses. Utilize a habit tracker app (the Apple Health app has a medication tracker you can use), use a paper calendar, leave sticky notes on your refrigerator, or set reminders on your phone for your injection day. It doesn't matter how you do it, but avoiding those inconsistent injections will help get you where you want to be faster.

112 Get Realistic with Your Weight Loss Expectations

A common trap you can fall into when you desire weight loss is setting an unrealistic goal weight. What makes a goal unrealistic? It will vary from person to person but a few examples are:

- If you haven't seen that number on the scale since you were in your teenage years, it's likely that wouldn't be a healthy weight for you now.
- If you haven't seen that number on the scale since before you started weight training and exercising regularly, it's likely not a healthy number for you.
- If you haven't seen that number on the scale since before you had several children, it's likely that even if you get back to that specific number you will not have the same physical appearance as before you had children.

Setting unrealistic expectations around a goal weight will only lead to frustration and resentment toward yourself, and can even cause you to develop unhealthy habits like intentionally undereating to try to see that lower number.

To set a realistic weight loss goal for yourself, think about:

- How do you imagine you will feel when you hit your goal?
- What do you want to be able to physically accomplish?
- How would you feel if you accomplish your physical goal, and feel how you want to feel, but the number on the scale doesn't match what you were aiming for?

You may be surprised to learn how positive your weight loss journey can be if you focus less on what the scale number says, and more on how you are feeling, and what you can accomplish!

113 | There Is No Weight Loss Guarantee

GLP-1 medications have changed the landscape of obesity treatment. With the intense promotion of GLP-1 medications paired with personal testimonials and weight loss journeys being shared on social media, many people who decide to take GLP-1 medications feel entitled to guaranteed weight loss. Here's a healthy dose of reality though: You're not entitled or guaranteed to lose any weight while taking your GLP-1 medication.

Keep in mind that your body doesn't care if you want to lose weight or not; weight loss is earned through work. You must create a safe and stable environment for your body to lose weight safely, otherwise you'll find it may not cooperate with your plan. Extreme calorie restriction likely won't do much for you other than allow you to drop some water weight short term and prevent you from losing fat mass. Pairing a GLP-1 medication with an inconsistent routine (regarding food intake, sleep, stress management, hydration, and exercise) can create no weight loss results at all. There are always exceptions to every rule, but for the average person, you will need to dial in your routines and habits if you want to see meaningful weight loss with your GLP-1.

To give yourself a better shot at as close to a guarantee as you can get: Create and follow through with a plan that includes your nutrition, hydration, exercise, sleep, and stress management variables. When you dial it in, weight loss should follow. If you are on top of all your habits and still see no weight loss on your GLP-1 and it's been over four weeks, consult your healthcare provider for support.

114 Set SMART Goals

You may have heard of SMART goals. It's a popular goal-setting framework, and it's important to apply this concept to your GLP-1 goals to set yourself up for success.

SMART stands for *s*pecific, *m*easurable, *a*chievable, *r*elevant, and *t*ime-bound in the context of creating a goal. The idea behind the framework is that the more specific you are with your goals, as long as they're realistic, the more likely you are to follow through and accomplish them. The framework also allows you to make adjustments to your goals if needed as circumstances can always change.

An example of a SMART goal related to taking your GLP-1 medication could be: *I plan to eat at least four small meals per day, each containing a protein source as the main portion, for the next four weeks to be able to increase my protein and calorie intake.* This goal is *specific* because it names the amount of meals per day with protein as a focus; it's *measurable* because you can check if you did have the four meals per day; it's *achievable* because you have the means to eat several times per day; it's *relevant* because you are trying to have frequent balanced meals; and it's *time-bound* because you will reassess after working on it for four weeks.

The following steps will give you a framework for implementing SMART goals into your life:

1 Audit where you are currently struggling and create a list of those areas.

2 Take your list from step one and identify your top two or three most challenging areas.

3 Draft a SMART goal for each area with a specific timeframe in mind to revisit your progress.

4 Repeat the process regularly to help keep yourself focused and making progress.

115 Start Small and Think Incrementally

A surefire way to get overwhelmed—and toss all consideration and care for your health out the window—is to take jumps that are too big or to take on more than you can handle at one time. A major pattern that can be seen in those who don't follow through on their goals or maintain their progress long term is that the way they went about obtaining their goal wasn't small or sustainable.

You're spending your hard-earned money on a GLP-1 medication and taking the time out of your day to optimize your lifestyle factors to have the most success, so be sure to set yourself up to maintain that success long term. Instead of jumping off the entire metaphorical cliff with an extreme plan or no plan at all, try breaking down your plan into smaller pieces and goals.

When you start with small goals and habits, it allows you to lay the foundation for habits to become routines. If you want to maintain your results and health improvements over time, the habits you are practicing need to become routines, so that even if life gets busy you're still able to maintain your lifestyle (for the most part) until things calm down. If you can't maintain what you did to get your results, your results won't stick long term. As you conquer one small goal at a time, or a few small goals at a time, you can build into bigger goals incrementally. As these goals add up and become more advanced, you are forming a routine that you should be able to maintain long term. Set the foundation, let it solidify, then build on top of it!

116 Lean Into Flexibility

Tackling weight loss goals or healthy habit changes requires patience and flexibility. The more flexible and adaptable you are when things get a bit off track, the better the chances are that you will be able to make healthy changes that last long term. If you can thrive and stick to your goals or targets only when everything goes to plan, chances are that you will keep falling off the metaphorical path. A rigid approach will likely lead you to disappointment, inconsistency, and frustration. Instead, create a flexible game plan you can tap into when life inevitably gets wonky.

The flexibility game plan framework is as follows:

1. Start by listing each goal or variable you are working toward (example: 60 minutes of walking per day).
2. Take each variable and create a backup plan to follow if your schedule or circumstances won't allow you to complete your initial target (Plan A: 60 minutes of walking per day; Plan B: 30 minutes of walking per day).
3. Break that backup plan into at least one additional backup plan (Plan B: 30 minutes of waking per day; Plan C: 15 minutes of walking per day).

By creating several backup plans for each goal you're working on, you can still make progress toward your overall goals by practicing your habits at different levels. Start with creating a Plan B and Plan C, and you can continue breaking it down more if you'd like, but eventually your last backup plan will be to let go of that specific goal for a few days to weeks until things calm down (which is completely acceptable if you have to take some periodic steps back). Barriers are bound to pop up to block you from executing your Plan A every day, so revert to your backup plans to keep your forward progress.

117   Learn What's *Actually* Realistic

One of the hardest parts of a weight loss journey is having realistic expectations. If you start with expectations that your weight loss will be instantaneous, you're probably going to be disappointed. Even with GLP-1 medication, significant weight loss will take time . . . and that's a good thing!

It can be hard to decipher what is or isn't safe for weight loss, but one of the best tips for a healthy weight loss process is to understand what's actually realistic and build your goals from there. Let's break it down: Healthy and safe rates of weight loss on average will range from 0.5–1 pound per week but can be up to 1–2 pounds per week, and potentially even a little bit higher if you're looking to lose over 100 pounds. That's your goal weight loss range per week, and if your weight loss is happening faster than 1–2 pounds per week, you should actually be focused on slowing it down.

Be sure to proceed with realistic and fair expectations in mind to support your mental and physical health as you achieve your weight loss goals.

118 Focus On Long-Term Habits

Long-term habits that focus more on your overall health, routines, and patterns are going to be just as important to develop as your short-term goals if you want to maintain all the hard work you're putting in while taking your GLP-1 medication. There's a time and a place for smaller goals and more specific tracking of your targets, especially during weight loss phases, but maintaining your overall healthy habits for a lifetime of healthiness requires you to be able to maintain routines. You are not meant to keep track of every single calorie, ounce of water, or gram of protein for your entire life. It's a great short-term tool to learn the different values of things so that when you are ready to maintain your health, you can put less emphasis on specifics and enjoy life without counting and tracking every single detail.

General habits that support your long-term health that you want to be able to maintain include:

- Practicing daily movement of some form (walking, stretching, structured workouts).
- Ensuring you're eating regularly throughout the day and not skipping meals.
- Incorporating daily stress management work to mitigate stressors (meditation, journaling, and so on).
- Prioritizing sleeping enough each night.
- Staying hydrated throughout the day.

For all of these habits, you can benefit from breaking them down and monitoring them more closely; however, your ability to prioritize and maintain these habits without having to put extra effort into them will be what carries you to sustainability long term. Practice makes progress (not perfection) with these habits for your long-term health.

119 Keep Moving Forward with Consistency

One of the most applicable sayings to your health journey, with or without your GLP-1 medication, is the saying "You are a reflection of what you do the majority of the time." This is the main piece of advice that anyone working on their health who wants to see their results last long term should take into advisement. In your normal day, there are always going to be things you won't be able to control. Most days your controllables will outweigh what's out of your control; however, life can get wacky and flip the scales without warning.

It's in these moments that it's important to remember that you can deviate from your plans for short periods of time and still keep making progress toward your goals. A couple days where you aren't able to be as consistent as you'd like doesn't mean that you have thrown all your progress out the window and have to start over. You need to ditch that all-or-nothing thinking. Rather, you are going to focus on what you can do to keep moving forward toward your goal. Gone are the days when you say you are starting over on Monday or are back at square one. Your health journey is one long ongoing road trip and you sometimes will take some detours, but eventually you can just jump right back onto the highway to health.

120 Track Your Progress

To keep track of your progress, you don't have to be a data lover or a fan of splashy spreadsheets to do it successfully, but bonus points if you like to keep it neat and coordinated. No matter how you decide to track your progress, it's important to have some sort of record to document how far you've come. When you are on a weight loss journey, especially with higher numbers of weight loss, you can become blind to your progress, which can turn into you diminishing all your hard work and how much you've accomplished.

There are several ways to keep track of your progress; how you do it should be based on your personal preference and how your brain likes to look at things. You can:

- Keep a spreadsheet of your weekly data points.
- Keep a paper sheet for major milestones.
- Utilize a journal to track your data points with color coding.
- Track digitally in a note on your phone.
- Use a check-in form and send yourself a check-in each week with your information.

When looking at what to keep track of, you'll want to keep in mind more than just the number on the scale. You can track your weight, calorie intake, water intake, physical activity, average steps per week, bowel movements, body measurements, or progress pictures. Pick and choose your priorities but try to have at least two to four data points that aren't related to your physical appearance.

121 Get a Clear Picture with Body Measurements

Taking body measurements refers to using a flexible, soft tape measure to get the circumference measurements of several parts of your body. This can be a helpful tool to see changes in your body composition during a weight loss journey as the scale doesn't always tell the entire story. It's possible to see little to no movement on the scale but have inches of difference in body measurements. When you're losing weight and resistance training at the same time, it's possible that the shift to your fat stores, water levels, and muscle mass can create a stalemate on the scale; body measurements can be used to get a clearer picture. There's also the possibility of human error with measurements, so inches shouldn't necessarily be the only measure of progress you evaluate.

If you decide to implement body measurements, here are some areas you can target:

- Chest
- Waist
- Middle of your thigh
- Middle of your upper arm (biceps area)
- Hips (widest part)
- Neck
- Calves

Best practices for taking body measurements are to use a tape measure that's specifically meant to measure body circumference, aim for the same spot on your body each time you take the measurements, and try to take the measurements first thing in the morning before having any liquids or foods. You can typically find the right kind of tape measure online or at your local stores. Be sure to keep track of your measurements in a note, journal, or spreadsheet so you can track your progress and changes over time as your hard work pays off.

122 Go Simple on the Digital Scale

Modern technology has given us the gift of digital scales and tracking apps, but they are not all created the same. Some come with a hefty price tag and promises of features that analyze your body fat percentages, whereas others give you a simple number and app for your phone that keeps track of your trends. With all the options available, what's the right one for you?

It's wise to remember that more isn't always better; sometimes less really is more. This is especially applicable in the world of digital scales for at-home use. Realistically the accuracy of at-home scales is only for the weight number that shows up. The additional bells and whistles that show your water weight, muscle mass, bone mass, or body fat percentage really aren't accurate enough at this point to be worth paying serious attention to or stressing over. Since you are just aiming to have the singular data point, it can save you time and headache (as well as money) to choose a digital scale on the simpler side. As long as it has a mobile app to go with it to track your data trends, it's perfect!

To get the best use out of your digital scale, there are a few best practices you can implement:

- Weigh yourself first thing in the morning after using the restroom, before any food or drinks.
- Stick to a regular cadence; weigh in either once a week or daily.
- Daily weigh-ins allow you to better see trends over time.
- Keep in mind that the scale will fluctuate daily, up and down.
- You are not defined by the number on the scale, nor is your success or failure.

123 Take Progress Photos with Purpose

Progress photos can be a controversial method of keeping track of your weight loss journey. Any tracking method will have pros and cons; however, progress photos can tread into the possibly tricky category of mental health. They can be an incredible tool to see major changes to body composition over several weeks, and when they are used with a positive purpose in mind it can be something to consider adding into your routine. On the other hand, for some people progress photos can create more opportunities for negative self-talk and potentially worsen your body image.

Here are some pros and cons of progress photos for you to see if they could be a good option for you during your time taking a GLP-1 medication.

PROS

- Help highlight overall progress over longer periods of time.
- Can show body composition changes even if the number on the scale isn't moving.
- Can highlight improvements to muscle mass.
- Can provide inspiration for self-improvement.

CONS

- Doesn't show great progress from week to week.
- Can contribute to negative body image.
- Can increase nitpicking or negative self-talk.
- Can be misleading depending on time of day, lighting, and clothing worn.

If you decide that you want to try progress photos as a method of progress tracking, aim to keep your photos as consistent as possible. Take them at the same time of day, in the same spot, with the same (or similar) clothing. You can have a friend help take the photos or use the front camera on your phone with a timer or video recording that you can screenshot.

124 Track Your Body Composition

While embarking on your weight loss journey with a GLP-1 medication on deck, a DEXA scan can be a helpful progress-tracking method. A DEXA (dual x-ray absorptiometry) scan is a low-dose x-ray scan and it's used as the gold standard for body composition testing. A DEXA scan looks at fat mass, muscle mass, water mass, and bone mass (density). This gives you an incredibly accurate analysis of the entire breakdown of your body composition and helps you monitor your fat mass loss and muscle mass loss so you can better control your muscle mass loss.

All you have to do is find a local business or university that offers it and hop onto the machine for just a few minutes while it does the scan. It's noninvasive and there's no enclosure of the machine, so no worries if you don't like small spaces.

To best implement a DEXA scan in your routine for tracking your body composition changes, aim to get a scan every three to four months while you're actively losing weight in a calorie deficit. If you're maintaining, every six months can be helpful to monitor for changes. You can usually find great deals on DEXA scans by googling "DEXA scans near me" to see specials.

125 Find Your Way with Fitness Trackers

From smart watches to activity-tracking bands to smart rings, smart fitness-tracking devices are all the rage these days. When determining if a fitness tracker is right for you, you'll want to think through if you have the budget for one (the cost of the tracker itself, paired with any monthly membership fees to their app) and if you have a healthy enough relationship with your health data to use it responsibly. By no means do you have to have any kind of smart fitness tracker to go along with your GLP-1 journey, but if you have the disposable income to buy one, and can use your data objectively (without judging yourself or becoming neurotic about it), absolutely go for it.

You can use these smart trackers to keep tabs on your workout performance and recovery, daily steps, and changes to your overall resting heart rate; to track your body temperature and menstrual cycles; and most importantly to get a look into your time spent sleeping and the quality of that sleep each night. The least invasive way to do this is to pick out a smart ring as it takes up little space and you barely notice it's there, but you can also grab a smart watch that you can get the same data from (but it can be more uncomfortable to sleep with). With the data from a smart tracker you can:

- Track your daily steps and adjust your step targets and goals more accurately.
- Monitor your time and quality of sleep to better understand your patterns and improve your sleep.
- Keep tabs on your heart rate and its average trend that can improve as your health improves.
- Understand where you're at in your menstrual cycle (if applicable) and how that impacts how you're performing and feeling.

126 Slow Responders Unite

When you add a GLP-1 medication to your life, you likely have high hopes and high expectations. You're excited for your health to transform and to finally feel in control of your weight or chronic condition. So you start your medication and wait to see success . . . but it's not happening. You're frustrated and wondering why in the world you are not seeing the weight loss that everyone else seems to be. There is some movement on the scale but it feels like it's slower than a sloth. So what's the issue?

You may be part of the unique and special group known as the slow responders. The hard part about GLP-1 medications is that while many people respond with steady weight loss (some even are hyper-responders who lose too quickly), there's a whole segment of GLP-1 users who are slower to respond. The reasons behind this will vary based on genetics, habits, environment, and health history. GLP-1 experiences can feel isolating under the best of circumstances, so please know if you're not seeing immediate results, you're not alone. It's possible that something you are or aren't doing could be causing you to respond more slowly, so to ensure it's not something you can change, be sure you:

- Are taking your medication as prescribed and not skipping doses.
- Aren't taking other medications that can interfere with your GLP-1.
- Have implemented all the lifestyle changes consistently (eating enough calories, protein, fruits, and vegetables; managing stress; limiting alcohol; sleeping enough; and exercising regularly).

Most importantly, if you find yourself in the slow responder club, maintain your lifestyle habits to support your GLP-1 journey and give yourself grace and compassion.

127 Make Sleep Your Foundation

If someone told you that lack of sleep was the reason you were struggling to lose weight, would you believe them? Well, they could actually be right. Sleep is absolutely the foundation of your health; one way to think of it is that sleep is the backbone or spine of your health journey. Everything depends on it. If your sleep isn't in check, in duration or quality, you can wave goodbye to your weight loss goal.

When you are chronically short on sleep, your body is more likely to hold on to your fat mass, directly working against you and your GLP-1 medication. Insulin sensitivity also drops when you aren't getting enough sleep, which is a direct slap to your GLP-1. In addition to the physiological changes you can see if you aren't sleeping enough, your sleep deprivation can also impact your decision-making. You are more likely to make poor decisions around food when you are lacking sleep.

So what can you do to strengthen your sleep and have a healthy foundation?

- Aim to start your wind-down routine for bed around the same time every night.
- Avoid screens or use blue light blockers for 2 hours before bed.
- Create a peaceful, distraction-free environment for bedtime.
- Limit excessive liquid intake right before bed so you're not up all night running to the bathroom.

128 Find Your Ideal Sleep Temperature

Since sleep is a critical component for successful weight loss, you'll want to set yourself up to get the best sleep you can possibly get to work hand in hand with your GLP-1 medication.

Throughout the day, your body temperature fluctuates, with your coolest temperature being at the beginning of the day and your warmest at the end of the day. When it's time for bed, as your body is relaxing, it releases heat to bring your temperature down for bedtime. The room temperature, your pajamas, and your bedding all can have an impact on your sleep quality, so it's important to create a comfortable environment in your bedroom. If the room is too warm it can disrupt your body's cooling ability. If your bedding or pajamas are trapping too much heat and preventing you from cooling down, even in a cool room, that can hurt your sleep quality.

According to the National Sleep Foundation, 65°F–68°F is the ideal range to promote quality sleep. Individual preferences will vary, especially for older adults, who may require warmer rooms at night. Or you may prefer cozy pajamas and extra bulky bedding, in which case you'd want to consider setting the thermostat at the lower end of that temperature range.

129 Keep Nighttime Reflux at Bay

Reflux is an unwelcome guest any time of day, but when it starts encroaching on your sleep, it becomes even more of a problem. You already know that as you are taking your GLP-1 medication, sleep is pivotal to your weight loss success, so reflux disrupting your sleep simply will not fly.

In order to keep reflux at bay, you'll want to be sure you are avoiding any reflux triggers you may struggle with so as to not put yourself at a bigger disadvantage. Spicy foods, alcohol, caffeine, and carbonation ideally should be tossed out the window or at least skipped at the dinner table. With these triggers out of the picture, you can also try to space your dinner or last meal of the day further away from bedtime so you can have more time upright to allow for digestion before bed.

Outside of food interventions, you can adjust your sleeping position to give almost immediate relief. Propping yourself up so that you're sleeping at an angle can help gravity pull down any rising stomach acids and avoid your esophagus burning all night. The easiest way to stay propped up would be to use a wedge pillow. A wedge pillow is essentially like a ramp that allows you to put your favorite pillows on top for comfort but also keeps you up at an angle for relief. Lying on your left side in general can also support digestion and decrease reflux; pair that with the wedge pillow, and you've got a match made in reflux-free heaven.

130 Explore Binaural Beats for Sleep

If you aren't sleeping enough or aren't getting quality sleep, that will work directly against your weight loss efforts, even with your GLP-1 medication. Lack of sleep can cause increased hunger, make you less sensitive to insulin, slow your metabolism, and can even lead to weight gain. Not getting enough sleep is a direct threat to your journey on your GLP-1 . . . but what do you do if you're having trouble sleeping *because* of your GLP-1?

If discomfort from side effects from your GLP-1 medication is keeping you up at night, try exploring binaural beats to help you sleep more soundly. There are two specific sound frequencies that can help lull you to sleep when you aren't feeling the best or are struggling to turn your mind off. Theta waves are linked to the early stages of sleep and lighter sleep, while delta waves are linked to deep and restorative sleep periods. When combined together they can create the perfect harmony of sound to help take you from alert and awake to deep sleep.

Binaural beats can be found on most streaming platforms where tracks have been crafted with two different frequencies to help you achieve the highest quality sleep. Look for an option that features theta and delta waves and try playing it as you're heading off to bed to let your mind relax.

131 Meditate Your Way to Sleep

With the major importance of sleep for weight loss and inflammation reduction, it's imperative that you are getting regular sleep at night, but many people struggle with sleep issues on occasion. If you're having trouble falling asleep or staying asleep, meditation can come in handy. Meditation takes practice and patience to see the full benefits of it, but if you can commit to the process it can really help with your sleep hygiene. When you are experiencing more stress, or you have something exciting coming up, you can end up amping yourself up, which interferes with your ability to fall asleep at your normal time or to stay asleep. Over time if this is becoming a regular occurrence, it can slow down your weight loss on your GLP-1 or even increase your inflammation. Your GLP-1 medication can only do so much; you have to work with it for the best results.

Sleep meditation can happen in two ways: mindfulness meditation or guided meditation. This will ultimately be a personal preference, and you should try out both forms of meditation if you are struggling to fall asleep. Mindfulness meditation requires just you and your breath. In bed, close your eyes and focus on breathing in and out, noticing how your chest rises and falls, allowing your thoughts to pass, and continuing to be centered around your breathing. If you're noticing your brain is still running wild during mindfulness meditation, you might enjoy a guided meditation more. These are audio recordings that give you directions on your breathing, what to think about, tune in to, and be aware of. You can find free audio meditations on YouTube, and meditation podcasts are available through most major platforms such as Spotify or Audible.

132 Battle Insomnia

When battling insomnia, you may need the help of your healthcare provider and medication, but you also may be able to beat insomnia without medication by using lifestyle changes. To find the best solution for your insomnia, it can be helpful to understand why you are experiencing insomnia (this can also help determine if you need medication or not). No matter its cause, recurring and regular insomnia will make it difficult to feel your best and see consistent forward progress on your GLP-1 medication, so it's important to not ignore it, and to proactively tackle it.

Insomnia can be triggered by increased stress, poor sleep habits, medical conditions like sleep apnea, anxiety, or even physical injury. To battle insomnia you should focus on establishing a positive sleep routine and creating a sleep environment that is conducive to high-quality sleep. To get the best sleep, ensure that you are:

- Establishing a consistent bedtime and wake-up time.
- Sleeping in a dark, cool, and quiet environment free from distractions.
- Skipping afternoon naps.
- Avoiding late afternoon or evening workouts.
- Not using devices that emit blue light (TVs, iPads, phones) for 2 hours before bed.
- Not drinking caffeine or using stimulants within at least 6 hours of your normal bedtime (some people are more sensitive to stimulants and will need to extend that caffeine-free period).

Prioritizing your sleep routine is your best bet for battling insomnia, and your body will have an even better response to your GLP-1 medication.

133 Investigate the Sleep Apnea Connection

The beauty of GLP-1 medications is that they are beneficial for so much more than obesity and type 2 diabetes. Zepbound specifically has been approved to be used as a treatment for moderate to severe obstructive sleep apnea in adults with obesity; this represents a groundbreaking treatment option for sleep apnea. Sleep apnea is a sleep disorder where you stop breathing multiple times per night. Obstructive sleep apnea can happen as a result of obesity, hormone changes, or even tonsil issues. You'll receive a sleep apnea diagnosis by working with your healthcare provider to get the necessary testing done.

How do you know if you have sleep apnea? If you're snoring loudly, find that you're exhausted during the day even with enough sleep at night, suffer from morning headaches, have a dry mouth after sleeping, have experienced unexplained weight gain, or have someone sleeping next to you that's noticed you stop breathing in your sleep regularly, it's important that you be evaluated by your doctor. This can be a crucial piece of your overall health puzzle to understand while taking your GLP-1 medication. If you feel like you're doing everything right but not seeing the progress you'd hoped for on your GLP-1, and you have the symptoms of sleep apnea, it's possible that you may need higher doses of your GLP-1 or if you're not taking Zepbound specifically, you may benefit from switching to this medication.

134 Don't Ignore Your Digestion

Digestion is the ruler of your life, especially when it comes to taking a GLP-1 medication. While that may sound a tad dramatic, you will truly have to place more emphasis on your digestive health while taking your GLP-1 medications than you would without them and that's largely due to the fact that most negative side effects or outcomes stem from your digestive system.

You're busy; you've got a life outside of your GLP-1 medication. You don't have time to read every single tip or trick that exists about digestive health, so you need a few pointers that you can implement without having to do a deep dive to find them.

Let's get right to it. Here are your digestion must-haves for your GLP-1 journey:

- Aim to eat breakfast within an hour of waking up and then a meal or snack every 3–4 hours after breakfast.
- Decrease your portions and increase the frequency of your meals.
- Avoid drinking large volumes of liquids before, during, and after meals.
- Chew your food well and take deep breaths before and during your meals.
- Try to walk 5–10 minutes after meals to get food moving.

135 Commit to Regular Mealtimes

You may be feeling the reality of no longer having a big appetite, and with a low appetite comes a higher chance of you skipping meals. That's bad news: When you skip meals, you not only are slowing down your metabolism, but you also can be creating constipation as a side effect.

Since you see motility and movement decrease in your gut as a result of your GLP-1 medication, you want to avoid long periods without eating during the day to promote regular movement throughout your gastrointestinal tract. One of the biggest keys to making the most of your time on your GLP-1 medication is eating meals regularly throughout the day. Regular meal intake while taking your GLP-1 would be four to six meals and snacks combined throughout the day. This supports your blood sugar and insulin levels, ensures your food intake doesn't drop too low, and helps you to have regular bowel movements so you can avoid constipation.

If eating more throughout the day seems like a monumental task right now, don't worry: This is a common response. To make a sufficient food intake more attainable, try breaking your overall calories into six blocks and making each of those "blocks" represent one meal. If the small meals you're having every 2–4 hours throughout the day still feel too big, try breaking them into even smaller pieces. Over time your body will adapt to the smaller and more frequent meals.

136 Say Yes to Breakfast

The saying that breakfast is the most important meal of the day may be a bit cliché, but when taking a GLP-1 medication, it's not wrong. With GLP-1 medications increasing your risk of nausea and impacting how much you can eat at a time, skipping breakfast starts off your day on a low note. When you plan for a balanced breakfast, you begin your day with a meal that supports your blood sugar, can reduce your nausea or eliminate it altogether, and helps get your digestive system going for the day.

Just because it's breakfast time, however, doesn't mean you need to eat exclusively traditional breakfast foods, especially if those are not foods you enjoy. Breakfast can be whatever you'd like it to be, whether that's a burrito, egg tacos, oatmeal, or a sandwich, as long as you have protein paired with some carbohydrates and fats, you're set! If your mornings are fast-paced and you feel like you don't have enough time to put anything together or cook, try making a smoothie packed with fruits, vegetables, and protein the night before and store it in the refrigerator or freezer overnight so you can grab and go in the morning. You can also prepare breakfast sandwiches or breakfast burritos in bulk ahead of time and store them in the freezer so they just need a quick warm-up in the morning before you head out the door (or you can even take them to work with you to eat when you arrive).

Bonus points if you eat your breakfast before consuming any additional liquids like coffee; this will help you avoid getting full before you can finish your breakfast!

137 | Get Your Protein Coffee Fix

Currently an Internet sensation, "proffee" is a protein shake and coffee combo, best enjoyed over ice. If you are struggling with lack of appetite, morning nausea, or protein-related food aversions, making a proffee can be your new go-to to start your day on the right foot. As you know, while on GLP-1 medications breakfast is a very important part of your day to support your blood sugar and keep your calorie intake up. At the same time, you know that with GLP-1s you may not be feeling hungry, can be experiencing extra nausea in the morning, and may be struggling with any food sounding appetizing. Now you can try proffee for solving these problems.

Realistically, almost every coffee lover tends to keep their morning coffee in their routine even if their GLP-1 medication isn't helping them feel the best in the morning. But with proffee you can hack your coffee and combine it with your breakfast. You can do this two ways. The first is to combine your coffee of choice with a premade protein shake. The second is to combine a protein powder with milk and add it to your coffee of choice. This combo is typically more palatable as it tastes just like your latte but with the added benefit of protein. While it would be best to have a more balanced meal for breakfast with some additional fruit or fats, a win is a win. Enjoy your proffee to kick off your day!

138 Limit Mealtime Liquids

If you're a habitual mealtime drinker to get your fluids, it's time to break up with that habit and create a new hydration routine. When taking a GLP-1 medication, digestion is slowed down; when this happens, your ability to break down food also slows down. Liquids during meals that are more than a few sips here and there can actually interfere with your digestive enzyme production, which can lead to you feeling bloated and uncomfortable.

No supplement can mitigate the impact multiple ounces of liquid will have on your digestion, so a good rule is to try to limit liquids right before, during, and after mealtimes. Everyone will have a different threshold, but approximately 30 minutes before and after meals can be a good starting point to test out limiting liquids around mealtimes. When you hear "limiting liquids" it might seem vague. To be more specific: Try to avoid having more than small sips of any beverages to avoid impacting your digestion. The small sips can be to keep your mouth from drying out or to help swallow if your food is a bit dry. Once you're in the clear after your meal, you can jump right back into your usual hydration routine to catch up.

139 | Stay Calm and Collected While Eating

While it's understandable that family dinners may occasionally make you want to toss your food at the most aggravating person in the room, your digestive system and nervous system would prefer you skip the food fights. Jokes aside, when you have a GLP-1 medication in the mix, it raises the importance for you to prioritize healthy digestion habits. Staying calm and relaxed during mealtimes is one of the easiest and most natural ways to aid digestion during meals. If you are eating in an environment where you are amped up, trying to fight with your tablemate (or even a phone mate), or yelling at the TV, that can disrupt your digestion and lead to indigestion and bloating.

To keep the vibes in check and be kind to your digestive system while taking your GLP-1 medication, try to:

- Eat your meals seated at a table.
- Aim to take your time eating through your plate.
- Avoid eating with distractions like your phone or TV on.
- Keep dinner company calm, or table heated conversations until after dinnertime.

Bonus points if you save the heated conversations until after dinner and discuss during a post-dinner walk.

140 Limit Highly Processed and High-Sugar Foods

With any discussion about highly processed foods, it must be acknowledged that having access to nutritious, minimally processed whole foods is a privilege that's not available to everyone. So while it may be best to limit highly processed foods, it may not always be possible. If that's the case for you, you can still make the best choices for yourself with the resources you have, and you can still improve your health with what you have access to.

Highly processed foods usually contain higher amounts of sugar, fat, and sodium; little fiber; and fewer nutrients due to how they're produced. Ice cream, desserts, sodas, candy, and fast food (burgers, French fries, processed meats) are some of the usual suspects that come to mind when thinking about highly processed food, but the category includes more than that. Other common highly processed foods include frozen entrées (pizzas, premade dinners, and so on), sauces, syrups, jams, chips, and pretzels. Just because they're highly processed does not mean that you can never have any of these foods, but you will want to try to limit them, especially during your GLP-1 journey.

Foods that are higher in sodium can impact your hydration and blood pressure, and high sugar intake can affect your blood sugar and insulin regulation, all of which can impact your experience on your GLP-1 medication and overall health. If it's possible, keeping highly processed foods to less than 10 percent of your overall intake can be helpful for improving your health in the long run.

141 | Pause on Digestive Enzyme Supplements

You may be familiar with digestive enzyme supplements; they've been around for quite some time. Digestive enzymes are proteins that help break down different nutrients. You have a natural production of digestive enzymes in your body already, with digestive enzymes in your saliva, and your gallbladder, liver, and pancreas as well. The enzymes amylase, protease, and lipase break down different nutrients. Carbohydrates and starches are targeted by amylase, protease and papain tackle protein, and lipase breaks down fats.

When taking your GLP-1 medication, you may notice that your digestion is different, which is to be expected. Does that mean you should take digestive enzymes? Possibly, but don't jump to it right away. Instead, start by focusing on adding more foods that have natural digestive enzymes like raw honey (amylase and protease), papaya (papain), avocados (lipase), and mangoes and bananas (lipase). You also likely can implement other lifestyle modifications before needing a digestive enzyme supplement. It's important to note that if you are struggling with side effects like reflux, vomiting, or gastrointestinal upset, enzymes are not a solution.

However, if you are lactose intolerant, the small intestine doesn't make enough of the lactase enzyme. This makes consuming products with lactose unpleasant because you're not able to break down lactose. In this case, a supplemental digestive enzyme for lactose breakdown would be helpful.

142 Manage Your Stress Levels

If you've ever heard the saying that stress is a silent killer, you won't be surprised to learn that stress can directly work against your weight loss efforts and can even lead to weight gain. Stress can drive up your cortisol levels, increase your hunger, and increase your cravings. When you're investing your money on your GLP-1 medication and spending time to stay on top of your healthy habits, you'll also need to manage your stress levels to reach your full success potential with your GLP-1. Unmanaged stress will work directly against your efforts and can even increase your run-ins with side effects from the medication.

When you're looking at how you can best support your stress levels and your stress response, you'll want to start by identifying the underlying causes of your stress. You may be able to eliminate some of your stressors, or reduce them, but there will inevitably be some stressors that you won't be able to get rid of. For those that you can eliminate or reduce, you can start with those intentional changes. Unavoidable stressors can still be managed through daily practices such as:

- Breathing exercises
- Muscle relaxation techniques
- Vagus nerve stimulation
- Yoga
- Journaling
- Calming music
- Nature walks

143 Try Breathing Exercises

One of the simplest ways to help support your body and its stress response is to implement breathing exercises. Breathing exercises don't require you to spend any money, go anywhere, or have extensive experience to do them correctly. They're a safe, quick, simple, and effective way to calm your body down, more specifically your nervous system. There are several different versions of breathing exercises that you can incorporate into your daily routine. They can be used in the moment if you're feeling extremely worked up or they can be used routinely for more proactive management of stress.

Starting with the basics, you can incorporate belly breathing. While lying on your back, place one hand on your chest and the other on your stomach. While taking a deep breath in, push your stomach out, then exhale through your mouth and your stomach should return back to the starting position. There's no minimum or maximum amount of time for belly breathing; you can try it for a few minutes at a time, or for longer periods, whatever you feel is best!

Once belly breathing is something you're comfortable with, you can incorporate what's known as 4-7-8 breathing. You'll start the same as in belly breathing but this time you will breathe in through your nose for 4 seconds, hold your breath for 7 seconds, and then exhale for 8 seconds through your mouth. You can try 4-7-8 breathing for as little or as long as you'd like; when you are feeling calmer, you can stop or keep going for additional practice. While breathing might sound simple, you'd be surprised at how long slowing down and taking deep breaths can go for helping your body feel less stressed.

144 Work with Progressive Muscle Relaxation

When you're experiencing high levels of stress, you may find that your body is physically paying the price. This typically will feel like sore muscles, poorer mobility, tense shoulders, and even your muscles feeling like they are extra heavy and weighing you down. Instead of letting stress take a toll on your body and in turn your workouts and your recovery, you can work to relax your muscles and your nervous system with a technique called progressive muscle relaxation.

This approach involves tensing different muscle groups throughout your body from the toes up for several seconds (about 5) and then relaxing them for at least 30 seconds. When you're intentionally tensing and releasing your muscles, you're helping your body activate its natural response to release the muscle tension that has built up as a result of stress. There are guided walkthroughs of progressive muscle relaxation on YouTube that demonstrate the stress reduction exercise, making it even easier and more accessible for you to incorporate it into your routine.

Pick your favorite quiet spot, take a seat or lie down, and get to relaxing those muscles. If you leave your tense muscles untreated it can increase your risk for injury, which can make a significant dent in your GLP-1 journey if you're unable to exercise. As a bonus, progressive muscle relaxation not only helps with managing your stress, but it also can be a useful tool if you're someone who struggles with insomnia.

145 Get Grounded

It's time to head outside to spend some time on the ground. Hopefully you've got some nearby grass so you can implement this new grounding technique to help manage your stress levels. All you have to do is head outside and plant your feet on the ground (in grass ideally, but any outdoor surface sans shoes will work) to ground yourself.

Stress management is an important part of supporting your weight loss efforts while taking GLP-1 medications. Stress acts as a direct hindrance to weight loss if it's not being controlled well. To some degree, stress is unavoidable, but thankfully there are various ways to manage it. Simply touching grass might be one of the easiest.

By going outside into fresh air, and ideally sunshine, you can bring awareness to your body and surroundings by physically grounding yourself into the grass. All you have to do is physically connect with the ground, skin to earth. Spend 5–10 minutes at a time practicing this technique to help calm your nervous system and recenter yourself so you can go on with your day newly refreshed and better positioned to be productive and practice those healthy habits. Research has shown that touching grass can improve your mood across the board and can leave you feeling a little happier than you were before.

146 | Stimulate the Vagus Nerve

Your vagus nerve, which is found in your brainstem and extends down through the abdomen, can help calm your nervous system and support your body's stress response while on your GLP-1 medication with a little stimulation that you can achieve through a few exercises.

When you're battling multiple stressors or experiencing higher levels of stress, your breathing tends to change, so calling attention back to your breathing and implementing belly breathing is a great place to start for vagus nerve stimulation. Gargling with water or belting out your favorite tune at high volume, receiving a gentle foot massage, having a laugh with friends or yourself, and plunging your face into an ice-cold bowl of water all can also stimulate your vagus nerve. In fact, there are multiple ways to stimulate your vagus nerve; in almost any situation, you'll be able to incorporate some form of stimulation to support your nervous system.

Not everyone will want to plunge their face into ice-cold water, but if this is something you want to attempt, you can submerge your forehead, eyes, and at least two-thirds of your cheeks into the water for about 30 seconds. It's worth noting that you may experience dry skin as a side effect of cold plunging your face; just keep that in mind so you can take care of your skin too.

147 Find Your Zen with Yoga

If you've ever wondered if there was a way to get your physical activity in, decrease your stress levels, and improve your mobility all at the same time, the answer is yes! Regular yoga practice can help you improve your mobility, counts as your physical activity, and helps regulate your stress levels and nervous system. If you have a schedule that's tight on time, having a triple whammy like yoga can significantly support your GLP-1 journey. Even if you are not crunched for time, yoga can be a great regular practice to add into your routine.

Yoga classes come in a variety of styles, from hot power yoga classes that will have you feeling spent when they're over to deep stretch and meditation style classes that will help you feel grounded, relaxed, and at ease. While these are two completely different ends of the spectrum, you can utilize all forms of yoga while on your GLP-1 medication. The faster-paced yoga classes can help with increasing endorphin production, which helps you feel calmer and happier. The slower yoga classes focusing more on meditation and stretching can help with reducing cortisol levels and centering your breathing, as well as helping you develop more self-compassion for your body and its abilities.

To find your Zen and get the most out of the benefits that yoga offers while taking your GLP-1 medication, you can add in one to three classes a week to complement additional forms of exercise. You can also make yoga your primary and only structured workouts and take those sessions up to five to six times per week with a variety of class types.

148 Journal Your GLP-1 Journey

Journaling is one of the most underrated forms of stress management. It's a safe outlet for you to map out and dive deeper into how you are feeling and why you may be feeling that way. During your GLP-1 journey you may experience heightened emotions, battles with your body image and self-worth, or changes to how people around you are treating you. A common experience during a period of weight loss, especially significant weight loss, is that you start to notice that people treat you differently when you are in a smaller body. In a society that ties worth to body size, experiencing the difference between how you were treated in a larger body and now in a smaller body can be jarring and hard to process.

This all can become overwhelming and hard to navigate without an outlet. Enter journaling. When you utilize journaling correctly (relative to your own needs) you can help lower those stress levels and improve your emotional regulation. To journal, you can pick whatever method feels best for you, either digitally or via paper. You can use prompts or just free-form entries to work through how you're feeling. Journaling is a way to talk to yourself about your problems, concerns, fears, and victories, and increase your positive communication with yourself. It can also help you process bigger emotions to allow you to reflect on the situation and what you can do differently next time if you wanted a different outcome.

No matter how you write it, journaling can help you succeed on your GLP-1 journey if you give it a chance.

149 Soothe Stress with Sound Baths

Your brain picks up on different frequencies that all serve different purposes. This is a fun fact that you can use to your advantage especially when you are navigating high levels of stress. By finding music that meets the specific criteria that's been noted to help reduce stress levels, you can create a relatively low to no cost intervention to help you relax and calm your nervous system. When you are listening to the right type of music, it can allow your brain to have alpha brainwaves that help you become more relaxed while still being awake, which is ideal to be able to calm down and still move forward in your day. Typically, music with about sixty beats per minute can link with those alpha brainwaves to start the stress reduction process.

This is sometimes referred to as a sound bath, where you lie down and are immersed with sounds. This can be done at home where you can be relaxed and enjoy a sound bath soundtrack that's been recorded to allow your brain to relax and destress. You can find hundreds of free sound baths online to immerse yourself in. To find the most success with incorporating music and sound baths into your stress management toolbox, be sure that you enjoy the sound of the music before using it to relax you (if you don't like the sound, you're not going to relax). Try out several recordings to see which you like and create a personal music bank to pull from when you need it.

150 Take Nature Walks

A beautiful, low to no cost, refreshing way to help manage your stress levels and the impact that stress can have on your body is to get outside and take a nature walk. The fresh air, the sounds of nature, the scenery of nature all can help lower your stress levels. This isn't just a normal walk or just getting outside, this is specifically finding an area around you that is surrounded by nature. If you live in the city, this will require you to travel a bit farther away from the city or perhaps you can visit a local botanical garden. Otherwise think about any local trails, open spaces, or parks that have been integrated with nature around them; they can all have walking trails or benches for you to take a rest on.

There's a specific reason for this walk to be in nature and not just a city block walk. Research shows that walking in nature can improve your overall health. Your brain activity that's linked to negative thoughts decreases after just a 90-minute walk when you're surrounded by nature. Your creativity, mood, capacity for empathy, and connection to the world around you all improve when you are spending time in nature. All of this is helpful in regulating your nervous system and creating a stronger metaphorical barrier that stress must knock down to impact you. Most notably for stress management, though, the scenery and views in nature support calming your nervous system by showing you calming scenes that help ramp your nervous system down rather than up. Even if it's a bit of a drive, getting outside for a nature walk at least once per week can be incredibly beneficial.

151 It's Time to Move

Everyone and their mother has probably told you that you should be exercising while on your GLP-1 medication, and they're right, but realistically you could not exercise at all and still probably see changes to your health on a GLP-1 medication. So if you can see changes without exercising why would you do it? Because, of course, you'll be healthier, stronger, and have better longevity with your health outcomes when you exercise. One other thing that everyone neglects to mention, though, is the nuance that can come with adding movement into your routine when it wasn't there before.

To create a brand-new habit with regular movement and actually see success with it, you need to start from the ground up. The thought of starting to exercise if you never have before or haven't in a while can be overwhelming. A new gym or fitness studio can be intimidating, and not knowing what to do at the gym for your workout can make most people abandon the effort and never get moving. To realistically start moving more regularly, you need to take some of the overwhelm away from just getting started. You can use these quick-start tips to help you get going:

- Try a few personal training sessions with a trainer you trust to get comfortable with form.
- Join a gym and only use the cardio machines for walking while you get more comfortable with the gym environment.
- Try out different fitness studios that offer free classes to experiment with different classes to feel out what you enjoy.

Remember that everyone starts somewhere, and the only person's opinion you need to worry about is your own. Move out of your own way and get moving into your new exercise routine.

152 Maintain Muscle for Your Metabolism

While you may be hearing from everywhere that you should resistance train, you'll actually be more likely to follow through on resistance training if you understand why it's important while you're taking a GLP-1 medication. Realistically, resistance training is recommended for everyone (regardless of whether or not they're taking a GLP-1) as you have better health outcomes as you get older and are less likely to have adverse health events if you've regularly stayed active. Specifically in the context of weight loss and GLP-1 medications, strength training is essential for helping maintain as much of your muscle mass as possible while the scale is trending down. The amount of muscle you have on your body directly correlates to your metabolic health. The more lean mass you have on your body, the higher your metabolism is, the more calories you burn throughout the day, and the better your insulin regulation.

By adding regular resistance training to your life, you'll be able to maintain the muscle mass that you currently have, and if you're not in a calorie deficit, you can even add more muscle mass to your frame. During a calorie deficit or weight loss phase, you will see the scale trend down, which reflects fat loss, muscle loss, and fluid loss. Preserving as much muscle as possible during these phases helps maintain a healthier metabolism across the board. The more muscle you have going into a new dieting phase also helps you have an easier time losing fat mass without a significant hit to your calorie intake.

For your muscles to work for your metabolism, try to do at least three resistance training sessions per week. You can resistance train up to five times per week to support your muscle mass and metabolism.

153 Establish a Regular Movement Routine

Let's walk through how to create a realistic movement routine that you can stick to while you're taking your GLP-1 medication and beyond. The first step is to focus on the key word *realistic*. If you don't start out with a plan that is actually attainable for you and your current situation, you're not going to stick to it. Be sure to take into account your current physical activity level, your current physical capabilities, any physical limitations from injury or your body weight, or any location limitations (no gym access, small home space, and so on). Then you can begin to piece together your starting plan:

- **Start with location.** Where are you going to be working out? Do you need to take into account commuting time to get there?
- **Pick your frequency.** Resistance training sessions typically take 45–60 minutes, and cardio anywhere from 15–30 minutes per session. How many times per week can you *realistically* commit to each? If you prefer group fitness classes, how many times per week can you make it to class? If you are currently doing no activity, start with one to two times per week and build from there.
- **Pick a program.** Find a program that matches your current fitness level and activity preferences. If you are a beginner in the gym, find a beginner program that you can easily follow while you learn.
- **Consult your doctor.** If you need exercise clearance or have other medical conditions that can make exercising dangerous, work with your doctor to find a plan that works for you.

As you become more consistent with your starting exercise routine, you can revisit and make it more challenging or increase the frequency as your physical capabilities improve.

154 Choose Your Movement Style

On your GLP-1 journey it's going to be optimal for your health if you can work with a combination of strength training and cardio; they're both extremely beneficial for your overall health, in both similar and different ways. The benefits of resistance training include improved metabolism, improved balance and coordination, improved bone density, improved blood sugar and insulin management, and improved external physique appearance (more muscle is how you achieve a "toned" look; you cannot "tone" a muscle). Cardio training also supports your blood sugar levels but in addition strengthens your heart, improves your sleep, improves your mood, improves your circulation, and improves your endurance.

Primarily you'll want resistance training for the muscle aspect and cardio for the heart health benefits. A major piece of exercising regularly, though, is being realistic with your time to follow through consistently. So, if while taking your GLP-1 medication you can only commit to one or the other, commit to resistance training. If you ever have a few extra minutes, add in some cardio; something is always better than nothing. Pair them together to become the best version of yourself, or pick what is most relevant to your current health status and physical abilities.

155 Have Self-Compassion

If you have a negative view of your body, it's typically linked with lower instances of self-compassion and positivity toward your body. If your patterns have typically been to make negative comments about your body like "I feel so fat," "I hate my arms," or "If I just lost weight I would look better," you likely do not have as positive of a relationship with your body as you could. By implementing more self-compassion into your routine, you can improve your body image and support your GLP-1 journey and the success that comes with it.

While taking a GLP-1 medication, it's more likely than not that you will experience weight loss and changes to how your body looks physically, which can worsen preexisting body image issues or create new ones. By practicing self-compassion you can help yourself navigate those changes with less negativity. With a more positive body image and a greater degree of self-compassion, you can improve your overall satisfaction with your health and lifestyle.

The golden rule of self-compassion when you're working on improving your body image is to stop your negative thoughts in their tracks and reflect on them. Ask yourself, "Would I say this same comment to my loved one (mom, sister, best friend)?" Chances are you wouldn't say something negative to someone you love, so why would you say it to yourself? You are responsible for loving yourself more than anyone else, and your body listens, so talk to yourself with self-compassion.

156 Take Self-Compassion Breaks

If you lean toward speaking critically of yourself out of habit, then you may want to work on improving your self-compassion while you're navigating your GLP-1 journey and the many changes that come with that journey. A self-compassion break includes three main pieces:

1 Acknowledging your feelings.

2 Validating that you're not the only one experiencing this.

3 Meeting yourself with compassion.

This kind of break requires nothing more than taking a step back from your physical or mental situation. You can implement this technique at any point because you don't need any physical materials or locations; you just need yourself. You can take those critical thoughts and work through them with self-compassion.

An example of where this could be helpful on your GLP-1 journey is if you are beating yourself up over the fact that you're not progressing as fast as you'd like to be. You can take a self-compassion break and acknowledge that you are feeling frustrated and as if you are failing on your GLP-1 medication. You can then remind yourself that not everyone responds as quickly as others and that there are thousands of other people who are experiencing the same thing you are. To wrap up your break, you can practice some positive affirmations and affirm yourself that this is your own journey that will go at the pace that is best for you and your body. You then can reach out to a healthcare provider for help if you want to see if you can do anything differently to increase the speed at which you're progressing.

157 Write Self-Compassion Letters

You're about to become your own best pen pal by writing self-compassion letters. As you know, if you practice more self-compassion in your life you are healthier mentally and physically. If you're lacking in self-compassion, no matter how much you can change on your GLP-1 journey it will probably never feel like enough and you'll continue to beat yourself up. By having a physical practice of working through your thoughts via writing, you can rewire those thoughts to incorporate more self-compassion and create a more positive experience for yourself mentally and physically.

When you create a dialogue with yourself through your letters, it allows you to change your critical inner voice and thoughts by bringing awareness to them, validating your feelings, and then meeting them with compassion. This exercise is going to be very individualized to your own personal thoughts that you're struggling with; there is no right or wrong way to write your letter. An example of this process could be to start your letter with a thought you have about yourself, like "I am ashamed that I let myself go" (bringing awareness to how you are feeling). Then you can validate in your letter that this thought is making you feel sad, embarrassed, or however else you may feel. Then to bring it all together you'll want to write to yourself with compassion that it's valid that you are feeling that way, and it's okay to be struggling with feeling this way, and focus on how you can improve how you are feeling without judgment.

You can use this either as a daily practice as you're increasing your self-compassion or more sporadically as you need it.

158 Incorporate Supportive Touch

When you're struggling with your body image or are having increased negative thoughts that make you feel like you're spiraling out of control while taking your GLP-1 medication, incorporating the practice of supportive touch could help. Supportive touch is a technique that can be used to help calm yourself down and feel more centered, and it doesn't require any supplies other than yourself and your mind.

Physical touch, whether from another person or from yourself, can be calming. In the supportive touch technique, you use your own touch to help regulate your nervous system. If you're familiar with oxytocin you may know it's a stress-reducing hormone that's made in your brain and sent into your bloodstream by your pituitary gland. Oxytocin is released when you practice supportive touch. If you're struggling to reset and find calmness, it can be worth a try; you never know when a simple lifestyle trick may help.

To practice supportive touch, you simply place your hands over your heart and take deep breaths for a few minutes. You also can place your hands on your face, head, neck, arms, or abdomen for the touch aspect and when paired with deep breathing you can bring awareness to your body and where you are at that moment. After several minutes, you'll likely find that your breathing has slowed as well as your thoughts. To successfully see progress with supportive touch, give yourself a couple weeks of consistent practice to see the most benefit.

159 | Explore Self-Judgment

Self-judgment during a weight loss journey paired with a GLP-1 medication can be a recipe for disaster and can be a major reason you struggle to view your successes as successes. Self-judgment means you are critical of yourself, your actions, your body, or your choices. Weight loss, and GLP-1 medications that support weight loss (sometimes rapid weight loss), can sometimes lead you to a self-judgment trap.

This could look like criticizing and judging how your body physically looks, or how slow the scale may be trending down. It can also look like comparing your progress against other people around you taking GLP-1 medications or being critical that you are taking a GLP-1 medication when other people may not need to. Blaming yourself for previous experiences that didn't work for you can also manifest as self-judgment. If you have found yourself saying or thinking any of these things, you're not alone.

Realistically though, what have these comments or thought patterns done to help you succeed in the past? Likely nothing except to make you less kind to yourself. Rather than continuing down the path of self-judgment, try to focus on exploring when this pattern shows up and work on redirecting through reflection. You can practice stopping your inner voice and redirecting it when it's getting critical. You can also try working with affirmations, working with a therapist, and, most importantly, working on being compassionate with yourself.

160 Seek Out a Therapist

Therapy is an invaluable tool for navigating major changes in life, and while taking a GLP-1 medication, you're likely to experience major changes in your life. Being on a weight loss journey is already a prominent tax on your mental health, but then add in taking medication for support, having to be very mindful and intentional about your healthy habits, and also balance the rest of your life in the equation; the challenges can add up quickly.

When you experience quick weight loss or significant weight loss overall, have a history of struggling with your body weight, or struggle with your relationship with food, it can pose mental challenges for you and your relationship with yourself. A common issue with weight loss if you don't have a healthy relationship with your body is that you can have a distorted view of your body so that no amount of weight loss feels like enough. If you struggle with food or food tracking, you might restrict your food intake to where it becomes unsafe. For many people, these relationships develop early on in life—but they can also potentially develop while taking a GLP-1 medication.

If this resonates with you, your best bet is to talk to a therapist to heal your mental relationship with your physical self. This will allow you to have a healthy relationship with yourself mentally and physically, and allow you to reap the benefits of your hard work and GLP-1 medication. To find a therapist who can work with you (insurance or cash pay), you can use the Psychologist Locator page on the American Psychological Association website (https://locator.apa.org).

161 Support Your Menstrual Cycles

Introducing a GLP-1 medication into your life can impact your menstrual cycle and can possibly impact your birth control. GLP-1 medications can affect your menstrual cycle in both direct and indirect ways. When you lose weight, your menstrual cycle can change; for most women, it becomes more regular and predictable. Then the GLP-1 medication specifically helps reduce inflammation and create a more regulated internal environment in your body, which also can lead to more regular menstrual cycles.

With GLP-1 medications slowing digestion down, and seeing fertility anecdotally improving, it's possible that your oral birth control may not be as effective. If it's taking longer to be absorbed while your digestion has slowed down, it's possible that your oral birth control may not be as effective and you could potentially end up accidentally pregnant. You'll want to use caution during your fertile window each month if you do not want to become pregnant.

To support a healthy menstrual cycle while taking a GLP-1 medication, the best thing you can do is track your cycle. You can use available apps, a digital spreadsheet or note, or good old paper to keep track of when your period starts each month to figure out roughly when you ovulate. For a 28-day cycle, most women ovulate around day 14. You can use that information to plan to get pregnant, or plan to use an extra form of birth control to prevent pregnancy. By knowing when your cycle is typically expected, you can keep tabs to ensure everything is happening as expected.

162 Create Your Vacation Plan

Who doesn't love a nice vacation? It's relaxing to get away, enjoy new experiences and new foods (or favorite foods that you like to indulge in), or even enjoy a few more alcoholic beverages than normal (piña colada on the beach, anyone?). However, all those things can be more difficult when taking a GLP-1 medication. Your tolerance for alcohol intake is typically lower, foods at resorts are typically higher in sugar and fats, and disruptions to your routine can trigger side effects while taking your GLP-1. So if your idea of a good time on vacation is higher quantities of food, more sweets, more fats, and more alcoholic beverages, you're going to need a vacation plan.

One option to discuss with your physician is if you can skip your injection before or during your vacation. This may be a fair option to consider if you don't want to worry about managing side effects while on vacation, but skipping a dose should only be done with your doctor overseeing the decision for safety.

If you decide you want to continue on your medication as planned while on vacation, you can keep these general points in mind:

- Limit alcohol intake overall and space out your drinking throughout the day.
- Increase your water intake if you decide to have alcoholic beverages to prevent constipation and dehydration.
- Enjoy your meals by eating smaller portions of the foods that may be higher in fats and sweets.
- Bring over-the-counter support for things like constipation, reflux, or diarrhea just in case.

Have a happy vacation; you deserve to rest and relax!

163 Lean On Your Healthcare Bestie

While doing it yourself can be empowering and a great educational experience, realistically your experience on a GLP-1 medication can be greatly improved with a healthcare provider (healthcare bestie) in your corner. This can be a doctor, physician assistant, nurse practitioner, or dietitian—you just want a healthcare professional who understands GLP-1 medications and who you trust and feel comfortable with. You may need your healthcare bestie for support with managing side effects, making dose changes, and monitoring your lab work, or to get help with your specific nutrition targets and goals.

You don't need to lean on your healthcare bestie for everything, but you do want to increase your chances of success with your GLP-1 medication by having someone in your corner. To help you find a healthcare bestie who you can trust and work with, look in your local area or search online (social media can be great for this but make sure whomever you find is an actual legitimate medical provider, not a coach or someone with certifications). When vetting someone, be sure to review:

- What their credentials are.
- How they specifically can help you.
- Their approach to GLP-1 medications and obesity treatment.
- How you feel when you interact with them (do you feel heard, safe, respected, valued?).

Once you find your healthcare bestie, lean on them for support, and know that you can build your own team of healthcare besties who will work with you in their own specialty areas. Dietitians are the experts in nutrition and lifestyle habits and managing side effects with nutrition; doctors, nurses, and physician assistants are phenomenal resources for access to your medication, lab work, and symptom management as well.

5 Transitioning Off GLP-1s

Your overall health journey is really only just beginning for the rest of your life; however, your GLP-1 journey may be coming to an end. For many people using GLP-1 medications to treat chronic conditions and chronic obesity, often they may need to continue on their medication long term, but that's not always the case. You can choose at any time to discontinue your GLP-1 medication. This chapter will show you how you can recognize when it's time to transition away from your medication and how to successfully navigate that transition while maintaining as much of your weight loss as possible.

You'll also learn how to troubleshoot the transition off your medication if for one of many possible reasons—cravings returning, insatiable hunger, weight gain—you're finding difficulty with the transition. Walking away from this journey, you'll know exactly what you need to do to maintain your results in the long run.

164 Know When to Transition Off Your Medication

For some people, GLP-1 medications are going to be lifelong medications, especially if they have underlying health conditions that predispose them to blood sugar regulation issues and insulin issues. For others, it's a short-term tool that can be used to treat obesity and achieve weight loss results. So, what's the criteria for coming off your GLP-1 medication? There's no formal checklist that says once you hit a certain milestone you have to come off, but you can use your own best judgment in combination with your healthcare provider to make your most informed decision.

Signs that you are ready to transition away from your GLP-1 medications can include:

- **You've reached your weight loss goals.** Once you've hit your weight loss goals, you may not need your GLP-1 medication. If you've been able to maintain your weight while on your current dose, you can slowly reduce your dose until you're off the medication.

- **You've found out you're pregnant.** GLP-1 medications are not recommended for use during pregnancy, so if you're expecting, you'll want to work with your physician to wean off your GLP-1.

- **Your lab work has improved.** If you were taking your GLP-1 medication to see improvements in your blood work and now everything is back to normal ranges and you've been able to maintain your improvements, odds are you can discontinue use and maintain lifestyle habits to continue your progress.

- **Your medical conditions are well managed.** GLP-1 medications can be used to lower inflammation levels and manage chronic conditions that are flared. If you've returned to a well-managed state, you can work with your physician to discontinue the medication.

165 What to Expect When Stopping Your GLP-1

If you decide to come off your medication for any reason, it's important to be prepared for what physical and mental changes you can experience. Here are some areas that can possibly change for you:

- **Hunger:** Your hunger cues will slowly start to return to normal after discontinuing your GLP-1. For some, this can present as food noise and a return to fixating mentally around food. Pay attention to how you're feeling and gauge your hunger before each meal.

- **Satiety:** Your fullness at meals will likely change and your portion sizes may need to be adjusted. When you started your GLP-1 you adjusted your meals down to account for slower digestion. As your digestion picks back up to normal speed, your portions will likely need to increase for you to feel satiated after meals.

- **Weight:** Weight gain is always a possibility if the medication itself was the reason you were maintaining. Some people who discontinue their GLP-1 medication do report some weight regain. However, those who put healthy lifestyle habits into place while taking their medication have success when coming off of it at seeing little scale movement.

There's also the possibility that you may notice changes to your heart rate and blood pressure when discontinuing your GLP-1. Typically, GLP-1 medications can increase your heart rate, so when you come off the medication your heart rate can lower back down. The opposite can be said for blood pressure; it is typically lower while on GLP-1s, so it's possible if you have battled high blood pressure before, it may return. Every body is different and the transition will be unique to your own body.

166 Try Reverse Dieting for Sustainability

Before discontinuing your GLP-1 medications, it's important to return your calorie intake to your maintenance calories in order to be able to sustain your weight loss. This is a major puzzle piece to maintaining your weight loss that most people tend to skip. Reverse dieting can help. The concept comes from understanding that when you drop your calories, your metabolism adapts by slowing down. It can't keep operating at full speed when you are restricting the food that keeps the fire going. By adding in small increments of calories every few weeks, you are able to get your overall calories back up to your maintenance calories.

This is a process that everyone should be sure to follow carefully and strategically to maintain their weight loss. However, it's going to be most successful if you complete the reverse diet process before discontinuing your GLP-1 medication. Once you're eating your maintenance calories each day without issue and it's been three to four weeks of consistently eating enough, you then can begin the process of discontinuing your GLP-1 and maintaining your weight. Consistency during the reverse process and patience will be the keys to success to returning your metabolism to a healthy spot while getting to enjoy more food freedom with higher calories. Remember, calories are not your enemy. If you want to be strong, if you want to perform in the gym, if you want to be lean, you have to be well fed.

167 Maintain Your Weight Loss

Maintaining all of your hard work on your weight loss journey with your GLP-1 medication is often called the hardest part of it all. However, if you were able to build new healthy habits that have turned into routines before discontinuing your medication, ideally it won't be a huge hassle to maintain. The primary driver behind maintaining your weight loss results is going to be continuing to keep your healthy habits in your daily life. If you decide to stop exercising altogether, change the healthy foods you're eating, and ditch the discipline you've built up during your GLP-1 journey, chances are you will not maintain your weight loss. Your time, energy, and finances (for your GLP-1) all went into your weight loss journey and you want to honor that effort and investment.

To give yourself the best chance of maintaining your weight loss after coming off your GLP-1 medication, try to:

- Increase your calories to your maintenance calories with a reverse diet and sit at your maintenance calories for at least a month before discontinuing your medication.
- Keep tabs on your sleep so you don't create weight gain opportunities from sleep deprivation.
- Maintain the same overall level of activity (feel free to swap up the type of activity though).
- Prioritize balanced and frequent meals throughout the day.

If you notice that your weight may be trending back up despite keeping your healthy routines in check, there may be something underlying going on that would be worth exploring with your healthcare provider.

168 Focus On the Slow and Steady

Hopefully, throughout your time on your GLP-1 medication when you were losing weight, you took the slow and steady approach and focused on sustainably losing the weight. You didn't undercut your calorie intake, you focused on protein intake, you stayed hydrated, you incorporated regular movement, and you got great sleep regularly. Essentially you built a supportive routine to help your GLP-1 medication do its best work. While you were prioritizing taking care of yourself and progressing sustainably, you may have experienced weight loss that did happen more quickly at times, but as long as you were eating enough, it's still sustainable.

If you're thinking you didn't eat enough or you know you averaged less than the recommended daily calories while taking your medication, there's a very good chance you undercut your food intake and are going to see some weight gain as you discontinue your GLP-1. This weight gain is necessary if you didn't eat enough when losing weight in the first place. After you spend a few months at maintenance, you can go back to lose the additional weight slowly and steadily to be able to maintain it better in the future.

Slow and steady applies for losing weight, but it also applies to the ending of your GLP-1 journey as you return back to life without your medication. You'll want to slowly come off your medication, steadily maintain your routines and healthy habits, and continue to slowly make healthy changes to support your health in the long run.

169 Decrease Dosages

As your GLP-1 journey winds down, so will your doses. During your time taking your GLP-1 medication, whether that's been months or years, it's likely throughout that time you increased your doses from your initial starting doses. Tirzepatide users probably started at 2.5 milligrams and worked your way up to your current dose. Semaglutide users probably started at 0.25 milligrams and increased from there.

If you've decided that you're happy with your current weight or improved health outcomes and want to stop taking your GLP-1 in the near future, it can be beneficial to slowly drop your dose over the next several months to weeks. Of course, you technically can stop taking the medication cold turkey without slowly dropping your dose down. The cold turkey method may be the right fit for you if you're on one of the lowest doses and haven't increased much from the starting dose.

On the other hand, if you're currently taking one of the higher doses or the highest dose possible, it can be helpful to gradually lower your dose so your body can adjust to slowly getting less of the benefits of the medication. When you stop your medication, you will see a reoccurrence in food noise as well as changes in hunger and satiety levels, energy levels, and weight.

If you're able to drop down your dose levels one at a time, it will allow you to have a more seamless transition and adjust to less and less of the medication in your system. By the time you're at one of the lowest doses, you should have your routines strongly in place to maintain your results long term.

170 Think About Maintenance Dosing

When you've achieved the weight loss that you desired or have improved your health and are feeling great, you may be thinking about discontinuing your GLP-1 medication. However, rather than completely discontinuing you may benefit from staying on a lower maintenance dose of your medication instead. This will largely depend on why you started your GLP-1 medication and what benefits you found made the biggest difference for you.

GLP-1 medications are used for the treatment and management of chronic obesity, so if you have struggled with chronic obesity, you may need long-term use of your GLP-1 medication to manage your chronic condition. This typically will look like taking one of the lower doses of your GLP-1 medication paired with the continuation of your healthy habits to maintain your weight loss. You can always try coming off the GLP-1 medication altogether and if you find yourself backsliding even with your healthy habits in place, you can go back on the medication.

To determine if you should try a maintenance dose or come off the medication, ask yourself the following questions and reflect:

- What did your physician recommend for you long term?
- Before you started your GLP-1 were you struggling to manage a chronic condition like obesity or another that caused weight gain out of your control (like PCOS with insulin resistance)?
- While on your GLP-1 medication have you found immense relief from things like food noise or seen other improvements outside of weight loss, like improved inflammation or improvement of other conditions you may have?

If you answered yes to any of these questions, you may want to discuss long-term maintenance dose options with your physician rather than stopping your GLP-1 altogether even if you've hit your weight loss target.

171 | Watch for Withdrawal Symptoms

When you completely discontinue a medication, there's always the chance that your body will experience symptoms of withdrawal. While withdrawal symptoms with GLP-1 medications typically resolve on their own, they aren't talked about regularly so it's important to know what you should be on the lookout for so you can notify your healthcare provider. Discontinuing a GLP-1 medication will go differently for everyone, but thinking back to how you felt before your GLP-1 journey can give you a possible idea of what life after your GLP-1 medication can look like. If you struggled with insulin resistance driven by PCOS with high inflammation, it's likely those symptoms will come back. On the flip side, if your symptoms were related to habits that you were able to change while on your GLP-1, you can have a better chance at not reverting back.

To be as informed as possible when coming off your GLP-1, keep in mind these withdrawal symptoms, especially the medically critical ones. The most common symptoms that can reoccur after discontinuing your medication are:

- Weight gain
- Changes to blood pressure (typically will increase)
- Increased blood sugar levels
- Increased hunger and decreased satiety

You may also have headaches, dizziness, or notice things like abnormal heartbeat, difficulty breathing, or even chest pain, which all can be signs that something critical is happening. You should seek out immediate medical attention and contact your healthcare provider for support if you experience any of these symptoms.

172 | Use Meal Pairings for Success

When your GLP-1 medication is out of your system, your satiety cues are going to change along with your blood sugar stabilization. Since the medication is no longer impacting your blood sugar response or keeping you fuller with slowed digestion, it's important that you create the best meal pairings to support your blood sugar levels and keep yourself feeling full. When you look at creating meal pairings that can accomplish both tasks at the same time, you'll want to start with your main star: protein!

Protein is a superstar for helping maintain a healthy blood sugar response. When it is paired with carbohydrates you will see a moderate rise in blood sugars after eating, which is the goal. Protein also is one of the main macronutrients that helps with satiety because it is broken down slowly and helps keep you feeling fuller longer. Fats are the second star in your meal as they also are digested at a slower pace so you can support satiety with healthy fats in each meal. When you are digesting your meal at a slower pace, you will see improved blood sugar responses and increased satiety. The third star of your meal is going to be carbohydrates. You can't live without them! While they are the quickest to digest out of all three macronutrients, they are still an integral part of your meals to provide volume and essential micronutrients.

You want to aim for every meal or snack to ideally have a combination of all three components (protein, carbohydrates, and fats), but if all three aren't possible for smaller snack times, aim for at least two of the three, which will help you stay full and maintain a healthy blood sugar response.

173 Satisfy Cravings

After discontinuing your GLP-1 medication, you may notice your cravings are making a comeback with a vengeance. While taking your GLP-1 medication, you may have gotten used to not thinking about food too much and food in general perhaps didn't elicit strong emotional responses or create cravings for you. Cravings typically are triggered by dehydration, lack of sleep, restriction, or lack of protein. Thankfully, you can put a pretty quick stop to cravings to make them more manageable with a few lifestyle changes.

- **Dehydration:** When water is in short supply, your body actually confuses dehydration for hunger and typically that hunger comes in the form of a sugar craving. Try to catch up and stay caught up on your water intake for relief.

- **Lack of sleep:** Sleep helps you make better food choices, so when you are short in this department, chances are your cravings are going up and your ability to resist is going down. Try getting some extra sleep for a few days to reset.

- **Restriction:** If there's a single specific food that keeps showing up as a craving for you but you are trying to avoid this food, chances are this tactic is backfiring on you. You can actually experience worsening cravings that can lead to overconsuming certain foods if you restrict them too much. Instead, try to have a small serving of whatever you are craving and then redirect your energy to a different activity.

- **Lack of protein:** When you are short on protein, it can create a lack of satiety and create more drastic changes to your blood sugar levels. These shifts can create stronger cravings that can be hard to resist. Try having a protein-packed snack before succumbing to a craving to see if you can find relief.

174 Movement Is Key

During your GLP-1 journey you heard how important movement was and created a regular routine with a combination of walking and workouts. Your ability to maintain your movement is going to continue to be a key part in transitioning off your GLP-1 medication. While the rhetoric around movement while on your GLP-1 is heavily focused on preserving your muscle mass, those regular walks or workouts also created a stream of energy expenditure that your body adapted to. Your weight loss results are partially due to that regular level of activity that you implemented, so it will be important to continue that movement. If you were to discontinue your activity altogether, this would create a significant change to your overall calorie energy expenditure, which could lead to regaining some of the weight you've lost and worsening lab work.

So to maintain your health improvements and weight loss, aim to stay consistent with your same level of activity at least 80 percent of the time. You absolutely can swap out the type of exercise to keep things interesting and avoid burnout as long as you keep the overall time and energy expenditure similar. Your movement habit that you worked on regularly while taking your GLP-1 now will need to transition to a movement routine for long-lasting success.

175 Foods to Add When Discontinuing Your GLP-1

Without your GLP-1 medication running through your body, it's likely that you'll want to make some adjustments to your food intake to account for your body regulating back to normal. One of the biggest changes that you may notice without your GLP-1 medication is increased hunger and the need for more food to feel full during and after meals. If you keep your food choices the same as when you were on your GLP-1 you will be doing yourself a disservice.

When taking your GLP-1 you focused on smaller portions throughout the day and more nutrient-dense foods that had lower volume because your digestive capacity was lower and you became fuller faster. Without your GLP-1 you'll want to focus on having higher-volume foods that take up more room and you can also focus on having larger meals again if you'd prefer.

Swap out your higher-calorie and higher-density foods that have lower volume for higher-volume options that still give you calories but take up more space in your stomach. Some high-volume foods to swap back into your routine can include:

- Fruits (watermelon, apples, strawberries, blueberries, blackberries, raspberries)
- Vegetables (leafy greens, zucchini, cucumbers, tomatoes, cruciferous vegetables)
- Popcorn
- Broths
- Greek yogurt and cottage cheese
- Eggs and egg whites
- Oats
- Chia seeds

To create more volume you can add riced cauliflower to your regular rice or even add riced zucchini to your rice dishes. You can also try eating more popcorn as it has great fiber and is a high-volume food. Incorporating high-volume foods can help keep you fuller longer and support your hunger cues during life after your GLP-1. If you're feeling a bit out of control with your hunger, evaluate your food choices and don't forget to check your meal pairings to make sure they're optimized.

176 Foods to Avoid When Discontinuing Your GLP-1

After you've moved on from your GLP-1 medication it will be incredibly important to limit certain foods or avoid some entirely if possible. Since you will no longer have the support of a GLP-1 medication to help with hunger or blood sugar regulation, you'll want to be sure that you're continuing to create meals and eating routines with that in mind.

While on your GLP-1 medication you may have used calorie-dense foods with lower volume to get enough nutrients in you without having large meals. Without a GLP-1 now though, you'll want to take out those calorie-dense, low-volume foods to allow for more volume eating so you will feel fuller and stay fuller longer.

Foods that are high in refined carbohydrates (white breads, white pasta, crackers, and so on), high-sugar drinks (sodas, energy drinks, juice), sweets (cakes, cookies, pastries), and high-fat foods like fried foods all tend to create a higher spike in blood sugar after consumption. If you regularly consume these items they can create high blood sugar and issues with your insulin production as well. Alcohol is also an inflammatory beverage that produces spikes in blood sugar and should be avoided or consumed very infrequently to help maintain your results from your time on your GLP-1. You absolutely can still have a treat every now and then, as you are a reflection of what you do the majority of the time, so a treat here or there won't break your progress, but be sure you don't make it a common occurrence.

177 Keep Sleep from Slipping

With the discontinuation of your GLP-1 medication, maintaining a healthy sleep routine to get quality sleep and enough time asleep will be critical to sustaining your weight loss. It's a well-known fact that when you consistently get insufficient sleep, you're more likely to experience weight gain.

There are several drivers that can cause this weight gain including your impaired ability to use your decision-making skills to make good food choices, changes to your hunger signals, and changes to your activity level. For most people, when they're not sleeping enough, they feel fatigued and tend to skip additional activities like walking or workouts, and they are physically less active, which can change their energy expenditure. When your sleep drops, you can experience decreased cognitive function that can lead to increased cravings and your inability to resist those cravings, which can change your food intake. Your hunger and fullness hormones, ghrelin and leptin, are also impacted when you shortchange your sleep, causing your hunger to go up and your fullness to go down.

With the discontinuation of your GLP-1 you may already experience increased cravings plus increased hunger and decreased fullness, so if you add in lack of sleep it can become a double whammy that makes eating right difficult to manage. Thankfully you can be aware and prevent it. Aim to sleep at least 7 hours or more per night and ensure the quality of your sleep stays high so you are rested and regulated.

178 Navigating Weight Regain

The first step in navigating weight gain after stopping your GLP-1 medication is to stop and give yourself a little grace and kindness. Your body is wonderful and keeps you alive and moving every single day. Second, it's valid to feel frustrated, sad, angry, or however you may be feeling if you are experiencing weight gain after stopping your GLP-1 medication. You worked hard on your weight loss journey. So how do you navigate gaining weight after stopping your medicine?

Once you are ready to make a game plan with kindness for yourself, you can start by looking at the big picture. Depending on how much weight you lost while taking your GLP-1 medication, and how quickly you lost it, it's very possible that you will gain a few pounds back after stopping your medication. This isn't necessarily abnormal as this can happen after any period of weight loss, but if it's continued, significant weight gain where the upward trend isn't hitting a plateau, there's typically something else going on. You'll want to do a full evaluation of what's changed that could be causing your weight to trend upward. Check to see if your:

- Sleep has decreased in time or quality.
- Food intake has increased or decreased significantly.
- Activity levels have changed.
- Medications have changed or doses have been adjusted.
- Stress levels have increased.
- Hydration has changed.
- Schedule has had any major disruptions recently.
- Emotional and mental health has changed at all.

You'll be able to have a clearer picture of what's changed by doing a thorough evaluation of your life to be able to correct what you pinpoint is off. If you can't pinpoint a difference, it's likely worth consulting with your healthcare professional for more help.

179 Identify Your Root Cause of Weight Gain

If your time on your GLP-1 medication is behind you and you're seeing the number on the scale steadily go up and your clothes fitting differently, you're going to need to figure out why your weight gain is happening. Without knowing what's driving it you're not going to be able to effectively prevent additional weight gain. The most common reasons weight increases after discontinuing a GLP-1 medication are:

- **Changes to activity level.** You maintained a great exercise routine during your time on your GLP-1 but significantly decreased your movement when you discontinued. (Quick fix: Adjust your activity level back to what it was.)

- **You're metabolically adapted too low.** You didn't maintain enough food intake while on your GLP-1 and your metabolism adapted to low levels to keep you alive, but when you stopped your GLP-1 and started eating more your body held on to the slower metabolism. (Quick fix: You need to do a slow and steady reverse diet and track your food intake to readjust your metabolism to your maintenance calories.)

- **Your underlying conditions are not managed.** If the weight you lost while on your GLP-1 medication was initially gained because of an autoimmune condition or insulin resistance, you can see those cause weight gain all over again if they are not managed. (Quick-ish fix: Determine if you can manage these conditions at healthy levels without a GLP-1 or consider long-term GLP-1 use for management to prevent a yo-yo cycle of weight gain and loss.)

While these are a few common examples, weight gain after discontinuing your GLP-1 medication is individual and can be very nuanced. For the quicker path to stopping weight gain, working with a healthcare professional can help you find your root cause quickly.

180 | Step Away from the Scale

Digital scales do not run your life, nor should they dictate how you feel about yourself, but sometimes those human emotions do get the best of you. In these moments, you need to send yourself to scale jail, which is a fun way to say you are taking away your scale privileges for a while to be able to regulate your emotions about the number on the scale better. Notice how the scale is mentioned as a privilege? It's because it truly is a privilege to have a tool for data collection purposes, but you lose that privilege in the short term (or possibly longer) if you are no longer using the scale for data points and instead are using it to set yourself up for some self-bullying.

If you are in a spot where you have come off your GLP-1 medication and are digging into why you are seeing the scale trend up, the scale may not be the best tool for you at that moment if you can't stay neutral about what it shows. If you can relate to any of the following, it's probably time for a short trip to scale jail:

- You're anxious or worried to get on the scale and see the number.
- Your mood is impacted depending on whether the scale went up or down.
- You're getting on the scale several times per day.
- You simply want to take a break from weighing in.

Take a step back, give yourself a hug, and come back when you're emotionally feeling better.

181 Keep an Eye On Lab Work

The beauty of being able to get blood work done relatively quickly is you can dive right into any potential underlying causes of weight gain after discontinuing your GLP-1. Assuming you built in healthy habits during your GLP-1 journey, didn't severely undereat to lose weight, and didn't lose weight too quickly, there could be an underlying issue some blood work can identify.

Since GLP-1 medications can be used to lower inflammation and regulate insulin levels and blood sugar levels, it's always a possibility that your weight is trending upward because of an underlying condition that's driving inflammation up. Chronic conditions like polycystic ovary syndrome (PCOS) may require you to stay on your GLP-1 medication long after you've hit your weight loss goal to control inflammation, insulin levels, and blood sugar levels.

Your healthcare provider will be able to order labs to help rule out if there's high blood sugar levels, insulin resistance, thyroid irregularities, or inflammation that's the underlying driver for your weight gain. They'll work with you to determine if you should restart taking a GLP-1 medication. If your labs come back without any glaring issues, you'll likely want to consider doing a full habit audit to be sure your activity levels, food intake, stress levels, and medications haven't changed and are creating unwanted weight gain. One additional lab you can have checked if you are going through a particularly stressful time: a salivary cortisol test can evaluate your adrenal glands and how your body is handling stress (high cortisol levels can lead to weight gain).

182 Try Habit Tracking

With the emphasis on maintaining your habits and routines after you stop your GLP-1 medication, it can be beneficial to implement habit tracking to help you stay on track. Habit tracking comes in many shapes and sizes and you'll want to figure out what version of habit tracking is easiest for you, makes the most sense to your brain, and is realistic for you to follow through on. If you pick a method of habit tracking that is wildly inconvenient for your schedule or is a continual frustration for you, it's not likely to be something you will regularly follow through on.

Habit tracking, at its core, is keeping track of each individual habit and goal you have in your daily routine and if you've followed through on it or not. For example, taking your morning vitamins, eating three meals per day, completing your workout, drinking your water, and so on are all habits that you can keep track of so you are able to see if you're on top of your habits the majority of the time.

Decide if you want to utilize habit tracking digitally (via tracking apps) or on paper (in a bullet journal, regular journal, or just regular paper). Then pick how you want to keep track of your daily habits. You can try coloring-in boxes, checklists, striking through your list, using stickers, or any other creative solution you can think of. If you stick with your habit tracking, you're more likely to follow through on your goals and habits to be able to increase your consistency and maintain your success after stopping your GLP-1 medication.

183 Stop Wasting Time with Willpower

Willpower is often used as a reason for why you haven't been able to achieve something. You'll say you lacked the willpower to follow through and hit your targets, or you lacked the willpower to resist falling back into your old habits. This could also be lacking the willpower to resist over-eating, or to get up on time to get your workout in for the day, or even to just say no to extra drinks when you're in social situations. The reality is that focusing on willpower is a waste of your time and if you are hoping to maintain your results of your weight loss journey or health journey, it is discipline that will have to rule the day.

There will always be the occasional time where you can be more relaxed with your discipline, but you are a reflection of what you do the majority of the time, so if you want to maintain your results after discontinuing your GLP-1 you'll want to be sure you can stay disciplined more often than not. Rather than hoping willpower will get you through, tap into your discipline and understand that you won't always want to do something but you need to show up and get it done anyway. Willpower will wane the busier you are, the more stressed you are, the more tired you feel, and at the end of the day it will let you down. Set yourself up for success and keep practicing that discipline.

184 Maximize Motivation

Motivation is the driver that helps you show up and put in the work to achieve your goals, and when you do hit those milestones, it feels like sweet, sweet victory. Motivation can be great when it's at its peak; it feels like you're on the top of the productivity mountain getting win after win. However, motivation has a major flaw that can impact your progress: It can fall just as quickly as it rises. There are natural fluctuations in your motivation levels because lack of sleep, increased stress, illness, or even your interpersonal relationships can all drop your motivation right into the dirt. It typically will return to a higher point as whatever caused the drop resolves, but what do you do when it's in the dirt?

If your motivation has smacked into the ground, you're going to need to rely on discipline until it makes a recovery, but also know that you can tap into the work you did when you were feeling more motivated. When you are feeling motivated you need to maximize that feeling.

You can maximize your motivation in two key ways that will help you when you are feeling a bit low.

- The first is to prepare extra meals ahead of time and put them in the freezer. When you are feeling the lows, cooking can seem like a monumental task, so in those moments you can reach into the freezer to grab a meal you have already prepped.
- The second key is to prepare a buddy system for extra accountability in those low moments. Phone a friend and ask them to help you hit your workouts, get your grocery shopping in, or get your cleaning done.

Overprepare your current motivated self so your future self that is feeling low will have extra support.

185 | Have Determination for the Long Haul

According to the Merriam-Webster dictionary, determination is "the act of coming to a decision, accurate measurement, firmness, or fixed intention." You made an intentional decision to take a GLP-1 medication on your health journey, and now you've made another intentional decision to stop your GLP-1 medication, and you'll need to carry that intentional decision into your post GLP-1 life.

Determination is a critical component of maintaining your routines, especially when things start to go wrong; your kids are sick, your spouse is sick, you are sick, work is stressful and frustrating, your dog ate your sock and you're running to the vet, and so on. It's inevitable that life will get difficult, and it will make it harder to follow through on the commitments you made for yourself when your motivation takes a hiatus and the stress rolls in. Enter determination, which is essentially how you can maintain your post GLP-1 journey results for the long run.

To utilize determination to continue your success you'll want to be self-aware and understand your abilities, advocate for yourself and hold boundaries, ask for help when you need it, get creative with solving problems that come up, and always keep in mind that you determine what success looks like for you.

186 | Transform Your Habits Into Routines

If maintaining your results from your time on your GLP-1 medication is a top priority for you, you need to be sure that your habits have become your routines before discontinuing your medication. For long-term success, the habits that you paired together to have sustainable success on your GLP-1, like staying hydrated, eating enough calories, tracking your food, and so on, will need to have become routine in your life.

Habits are essentially tasks or goals that you are continually putting time, effort, and intention into on a daily basis. They can be easily derailed and distracted from, unless they become a routine. Routines are fixed patterns and behaviors in your daily life that even with disruption or distractions around you almost always still find a way to be completed.

A good way to illustrate how habits become routines is to look at your morning coffee or tea. If you have your caffeine every single day as part of your morning routine, even if your morning has been chaotic and derailed, you will almost always still grab your coffee. You didn't always have morning caffeine as a routine; it started as a habit and eventually became second nature. That's the same principle you will want to take over with your healthy lifestyle habits.

Routines are created with continued practice reps, intentional action, and awareness of your habits. Eventually the healthy habits you worked on or are working on from your GLP-1 journey will become more second nature so even the busiest of mornings won't completely derail you. Drinking your water or tracking your food will eventually become so routine that it'll be a part of your day without you even thinking about it. Remember, practice makes progress, so keep practicing to maintain your weight loss after your GLP-1 journey comes to an end.

Additional Resources

When looking for information on GLP-1 medications, it's critical to find information from trusted, legitimate, evidence-backed sources. In the world of social media, misinformation runs rampant, especially around GLP-1 medications. Following here you will find resources from other experts in the GLP-1 field to assist you on your GLP-1 journey. Whether you enjoy learning by audio or are a visual learner, there's a resource for you here.

🌐 Websites

Nutrition and GLP-1s

➤ **www.ama-assn.org/delivering-care/public-health/age-glp-1-agonists-food-choices-still-matter-health**
Information about GLP-1 medications and food choices from the American Medical Association.

➤ **www.glp1girlie.com**
Free educational resources from the author, registered dietitian Gianna Beasley.

➤ **https://substack.com/@summerthedietitian**
Free nutritional education from Summer Kessel, GLP-1 expert and registered dietitian.

➤ **https://thesleeveddietitian.com**
Resources about GLP-1 medications after bariatric surgery from registered dietitian Jamie Mills.

Educational Resources

✈ **https://my.clevelandclinic.org/health/treatments/13901-glp-1-agonists**
Basics of GLP-1 education from the Cleveland Clinic.

✈ **https://cme.bu.edu/glp1penteaching**
Links to video guides to using your GLP-1 pens from Boston University.

✈ **https://diabetesjournals.org/clinical/article/40/3/265/147056/Optimizing-the-Use-of-Glucagon-Like-Peptide-1**
In-depth education on GLP-1s for type 2 diabetes from the American Diabetes Association.

✈ **https://diatribe.org/diabetes-medications/glp-1-agonists-2-daily-injections-1-week-and-beyond**
The progression of GLP-1 medications from The diaTribe Foundation.

✈ **https://diatribe.org/diabetes-management/combining-glp-1s-cgm-improved-type-2-diabetes-care**
Research on combining GLP-1 medications with continuous glucose monitors for type 2 diabetes.

✈ **https://drspencer.com**
Dr. Spencer Nadolsky specializes in obesity and GLP-1s.

✈ **www.mayoclinic.org/diseases-conditions/type-2-diabetes/expert-answers/byetta/faq-20057955**
Understanding GLP-1s and side effects from the Mayo Clinic.

✈ **www.onthepen.com**
Up-to-date news on GLP-1 medications.

✈ **www.wegovy.com/about-wegovy/how-wegovy-works.html**
Wegovy information from Novo Nordisk.

✈ **https://zepbound.lilly.com/what-is-zepbound?section=how-zepbound-works**
Zepbound information from Eli Lilly.

🎙️ Podcasts

🚀 **https://drspencer.com/podcast**
Docs Who Lift *podcast from obesity specialists.*

🚀 **https://gamechanginghealth.buzzsprout.com**
GLP-1–focused support from the Game-Changing Health *podcast with dietitian Gianna Beasley.*

🚀 **https://onthepen.buzzsprout.com**
GLP-1 news and updates from On The Pen.

🔗 Other

📖 *Decoding GLP-1: A Guide for Friends and Family of Those On The Pen* **by Dave Knapp**
This guide provides guidance and a realistic look at what it's like to take a GLP-1 medication. It is a great read for family and friends to understand the GLP-1 journey, as well as a look into other stories of GLP-1 journeys. By the host of the On The Pen *podcast.*

🚀 **https://apps.apple.com/us/app/shotsy-glp-1-shot-tracker/ id6499510249**
Shotsy, an injection-tracking app developed for GLP-1s.

Index

About the Author

Gianna Beasley is a registered dietitian specializing in helping women navigate the world of GLP-1 medications by sharing a mixture of her own experiences with the medication and up-to-date science and research. Her goal is to help her clients feel empowered and supported—to create personalized plans that address their nutritional needs and help them make their way through their GLP-1 experiences with ease. Learn more at GiannaBeasley.com.

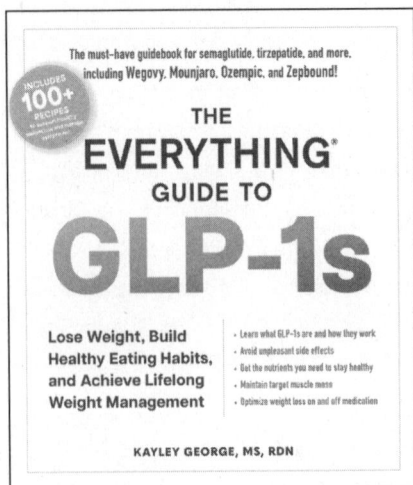

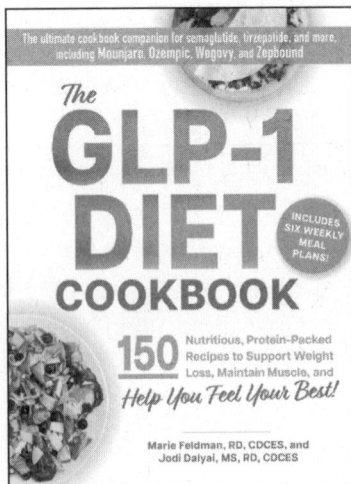